Oliver Sacks'

Awakenings

『レナードの朝』で学ぶ医療問題とクリティカル・シンキング

―Understanding Medical Issues: A Focus on Critical Thinking―

平井 清子　編著

NAN'UN-DO

このテキストの音声を無料で視聴（ストリーミング）・ダウンロードできます。自習用音声としてご活用ください。
以下のサイトにアクセスしてテキスト番号で検索してください。

https://nanun-do.com　　テキスト番号 [**511765**]

※ 無線LAN（WiFi）に接続してのご利用を推奨いたします。
※ 音声ダウンロードはZipファイルでの提供になります。
　お使いの機器によっては別途ソフトウェア（アプリケーション）の導入が必要となります。

Awakenings 音声ダウンロードページは
左記のQRコードからもご利用になれます。

AWAKENINGS ©1973, 1976, 1987, 1983, 1987, 1990, Oliver Sacks
by arrangement through The Sakai Agency

は じ め に

　『レナードの朝』は、実在の精神科医であり作家でもあるオリバー・サックスが、自らの臨床経験に基づいて書いた小説です。1960年代から80年代にかけて、アメリカのニューヨーク州、マウントカーメル病院で、脳炎後症候群を患う患者たちと、その治療に向き合った人々の物語です。
　ここでは、人間の尊厳と病気の治療のあり方という、現代の医学において課題となっている問題のほか、治験、そして、治療とそれを受ける患者の環境や心理状態に関わるテーマが扱われています。さらに、患者と治療従事者との関係、患者と家族の関係など、提示される課題は尽きません。その他、現代を悩ます「感染症」も物語の重要なテーマです。これらの医療問題を理解し、考えると同時に、これらに関する重要な用語や表現などの医療英語を習得していきましょう。
　この作品は1990年に、ロバート・デ・ニーロと今は亡きロビン・ウイリアムズの主演によって映画化され、その映画の製作にサックス博士自身が携わったことで、よりその完成度を高めたものです。その原作である『レナードの朝』は学生が英語で読むには難しいですが、その内容は映画では味わえない詳しい治療の経緯が語られ、また、様々な人間関係が丁寧に描かれ、全体に一貫して流れるヒューマニズムが読む者の心を打つ秀作です。さらに医療英語の自然な表現、重要語句などが随所に置かれ、医療を志す者にとっては、一度は読みたい作品でしょう。
　テキスト作成は、編著者が自ら教鞭をとる医療系大学の学生のために、この作品の映画と原作を用いながら手作りの教材を使用しはじめたことから始まります。この度、出版の機会を得て、学生の皆さんに分かりやすいように原作の英文を平易な英語に書きなおし、医療英語として必要な表現や語句を学習できるように工夫しました。さらにサックス博士の原書の中の表現を一部そのまま使用し、臨場感を味わいながら学習できるように配慮しました。その他、作品の中で提示されている医療問題を考える場を提供し、英語で批判的思考力（critical thinking）を培う試みをおこないました。また、この作品中扱われるアメリカの医療と生活に関わる知識を、各章に日本語でコラム形式で配置しました。
　幸い、サックス博士にはこの教材の日本での出版の意義をご理解いただき、版権を得ることができました。さらにご多忙の中を、全ての原稿に直接目を通していただき、いくつかの医学用語の適切な使用について貴重なご助言をいただきましたことに心より感謝申し上げます。
　本書が医学、薬学、看護、医療・福祉の分野など、将来医療に携わることになる学生の皆さんの英語学習に少しでも役に立つことができるのでしたら門外の喜びです。

　本書は2016年4月に南雲堂より再版していただくことになりました。再版での大きな特徴は、この作品を通して現代の身近な医療問題を学生の皆さんに英語の資料を調べながら"critical"に考える場を設けたことです。自らの意見を英語で表現することに是非チャレンジしてください。
　実は丁度その校正作業をしている最中の2015年9月初め、サックス博士の訃報が入ってまいりました。人間の脳と心の働きを解き明かそうと、常に人間に寄り添ってきた博士に心からのご冥福をお祈り申し上げます。そして、本書が博士の作品を一人でも多くの学生が読むきっかけとなるのでしたらこの上のない幸せです。
　最後に、再版にあたってはいつもながら貴重なご助言とご協力を賜った、株式会社南雲堂の営業部・岡崎まち子氏、加藤敦氏に感謝の言葉を申し上げます。

編著者

CONTENTS

はじめに …………………………………………………………………… 3
各章の構成と使い方 ……………………………………………………… 5
本書で学べる主な医療用語や医療トピックス ………………………… 6

■ Prologue

Chapter 1　　Life at Mount Carmel (1) ……………………………… 9
Chapter 2　　Life at Mount Carmel (2) ……………………………… 16

■ Awakenings

Chapter 3　　Leonard L. (1) ………………………………………… 22
Chapter 4　　Leonard L. (2) ………………………………………… 28
Chapter 5　　Leonard L. (3) ………………………………………… 35
Chapter 6　　Rose R. ………………………………………………… 42
Chapter 7　　Hester Y. (1) …………………………………………… 49
Chapter 8　　Hester Y. (2) …………………………………………… 55
Chapter 9　　Rolando P. ……………………………………………… 62
Chapter 10　 Miriam H. ……………………………………………… 69

■ Epilogue

Chapter 11　 Leonard L. ……………………………………………… 76
Chapter 12　 Rose R. and Hester Y. ………………………………… 83
Chapter 13　 Rolando P. and Miriam H. …………………………… 90
Chapter 14　 The Movie AWAKENINGS …………………………… 97

各章の構成と使い方

　各章（5～6ページ）は、以下の構成になっています。使い方や授業での配分時間を記載しましたので、それらを参考にしていただければ幸いです。なお、各章のはじめに日本語のあらすじやポイントが書かれています。最終章では、映画との比較をしています。時期は問わず映画を見ることで、さらに深い理解ができることでしょう。

　なお、Ⅶ・Ⅷについては発展学習として用意しました。学生の皆さんの興味や授業の進度に合わせ、適宜使用していただければ幸いです。

Ⅰ　PRE-READING（10分）

　その章で扱われる用語や、内容に関係するアメリカの医療、そして背景知識などについて、簡単なクイズ形式や説明などで英語で導入します。なお、ここで英語で取り上げられたものの中でも重要な用語については、再び他の章のⅥで、今度は日本語で取り上げているので、確認して学ぶことができます。

Ⅱ　VOCABULARY &IDIOMATIC EXPRESSIONS（15分）

　ⅢのSTORYで扱う用語を中心に、重要語句の習得をします。各語（句）の意味となる日本語、そして英語の説明文をそれぞれ選びます。

Ⅲ　COMPREHENSION（30分）

　STORYでその章の内容を平易な英文でまとめました。Notesを参考に内容を正確に理解するようにしましょう。CDを使って、聞き取りや音読の練習もしてください。次に、内容把握問題として、True/False Questionsが用意されています。これによって、内容をより正確に理解できるでしょう。

Ⅳ　USEFUL EXPRESSIONS（20分）

　原作の中で使われている、オーセンティックな英語の表現から、医療にかかわる基本的、かつ重要な表現を取り上げました。語（句）のヒントを参考にして、自分で日本語に訳してみましょう。本物の医療英語の習得ができる、このテキストの重要なセクションの一つです。

Ⅴ　LISTENING FOCUS（15分）

　原作の中で使われている台詞などを利用したダイアローグを作成しました。CDを聞きながら（　）に単語を書き入れましょう。また内容を確認しましょう。

Ⅵ　MORE ABOUT AMERICAN HEALTH ISSUES（5分）

　その章に関係した、アメリカの医療システムや病気、医療の歴史などを中心に、日本と比較しながら、コラム形式で日本語で紹介しました。他の章のⅠですでに取り上げられたものについて、より深く理解することができるでしょう。

《発展》
Ⅶ　YOUR OPINIONS

その章で学習した内容について、登場人物の関係や、一般的な医療問題に関する英文の質問を用意しました。英語や日本語で答えてみましょう。グループでディスカッションをするのもよいでしょう。さらに、英文で短いエッセイにまとめるなどの課題としても使用できます。

Ⅷ　MEDICAL ENGLISH ENHANCER（英語で調べてみよう）

その章に関係した医療英語の key terms を英語の資料で調べてみましょう。日本の事情と比較することで、より深い内容が学べるはずです。

本書で学べる主な医療用語や医療トピックス

	Ⅰ. Pre-reading（英語で）	Ⅵ. More about American Health Issues（日本語で）
Chapter 1	Encephalitis Lethargica（嗜眠性脳炎）	精神病医療の歴史
Chapter 2	Bronx について	嗜眠性脳炎とは
Chapter 3	Experimental Drugs（実験段階の薬の使用）	Parkinson 病と Parkinson 症候群
Chapter 4	L-dopa（L-ドーパの効用と副作用）	実験段階の薬と治験
Chapter 5	Amantadine（アマンタジンの効用と副作用）	アメリカの病院 (1)
Chapter 6	Psychiatric Care Team-members（精神科病棟で働く人々）	アメリカの病院 (2)
Chapter 7	Absence Epilepsy（欠神癲癇）	言語聴覚士（言語療法士）と視能訓練士
Chapter 8	Tic-like Movements（チック）	理学療法士と作業療法士
Chapter 9	Euthanasia（安楽死）	アメリカにおける看護師
Chapter 10	US Psychiatric Institutions（アメリカの精神病医療の歴史）	アメリカにおける医師と病院の関係
Chapter 11	Parkinson's Disease（パーキンソン病）	安楽死

Chapter 12	Clinical Trials（治験）	アメリカの医療保険制度
Chapter 13	Neurological Infections （神経系感染症）	アメリカ障害者法とは
Chapter 14	Useful Medical Terminology 病気の症状についての用語、薬の形態に関する用語	

Prologue

Chapter 1

Life at Mount Carmel (1)

　この話の舞台である、マウント・カーメル病院は、当時はどんな病院だったのでしょう。登場人物の紹介を中心に、そこでの生活やそれぞれの患者たちを襲った嗜眠性脳炎について紹介します。

Ⅰ PRE-READING

Encephalitis Lethargica （嗜眠性脳炎）

Have you ever heard of encephalitis lethargica?

Fact 1: In acute cases, patients may fall into a coma-like state.
Fact 2: The first outbreak was reported in Vienna in 1916-17.
Fact 3: Between 1917 and 1927, an epidemic of this encephalitis spread throughout the world, but few new cases were reported after the 1940s.
Fact 4: Some encephalitis-afflicted patients from the 1920s were still hospitalized, in a trance-like state, in the 1960s.
Fact 5: Even today, very little is known about the causes of the disease.
Fact 6: This disease may be characterized by high fever, headache, double vision, delayed physical and mental responses, and lethargy.
Fact 7: Post-enchephalitic Parkinson's disease may develop after a bout of encephalitis—sometimes even as long as years after disease onset.

Ⅱ VOCABULARY & IDIOMATIC EXPRESSIONS

The following terms are used in the story below. Match each of the following words or phrases (①－⑥) with the correct definitions (meaning 'in context') from the box below (a－f). Also choose the appropriate Japanese translation (ア－カ) for each term.

下の語（句）は、すべて **STORY** に出てくるものです。それぞれの英語の説明として、ふさわしいものを a～f の中から選びなさい。さらにその日本語の意味として、最もふさわしいものをア～カの中から選びなさい。

① motionless　　（　）（　）　② institution　　　　（　）（　）
③ kinship　　　　（　）（　）　④ against great odds（　）（　）
⑤ colleague　　　（　）（　）　⑥ debilitate　　　　（　）（　）

a) to make somebody's body or mind weaker
b) not moving at all
c) a large building where old people, orphans, prisoners, people who are mentally ill etc. live and are taken care of by an official organization
d) a strong relationship between people who may or may not be part of the same family
e) a word representing someone you work with, used especially by professional people
f) in spite of many severe difficulties

ア 困難をものともせず　　　イ （精神病院・孤児院・養老院などの）施設
ウ 同僚　　　　　　　　　　エ 親近感、一体感
オ 動かない、不動の　　　　カ （人・体を）弱らせる、衰弱させる

III COMPREHENSION

The following story will help you to understand life at Mount Carmel. Please read and answer the true or false questions below.

次の英文を読んで、正しいものにはT，間違っているものにはFをつけましょう。

STORY

This is the true story of Dr. Oliver Sacks, a well known neurologist, and a group of patients that had fallen into a sleep-like state in the 1920s and '30s. Dr. Sacks tried, against great odds, to 'awaken' these patients from their trance-like state. These patients suffered from 'sleeping sickness,' formally called encephalitis lethargica, a poorly understood disease suspected to be caused by a virus which attacks the brain and other parts of the nervous system. Although this debilitating disease had spread mysteriously throughout the world between 1917 and 1927, killing a third of those afflicted, many patients seemed to recover completely. However, many of these survivors developed 'post-encephalitic syndromes.' These syndromes are a collection of neurological and psychiatric disorders, most commonly parkinsonism, and these particular patients presented with very variable courses and patterns. In the late 1960s, one particular group of these post-encephalitic (PE) patients remained hospitalized in Mount Carmel Hospital in New York City.

In 1966, when Dr. Oliver Sacks first went to Mount Carmel Hospital, there were still some eighty PE patients there, comprising the largest known, and perhaps the only, such group remaining within the United States. Indeed, these patients, together with a similar community in Highlands Hospital, England, may have been among the last few such afflicted individuals remaining in the world at that time.

Between 1966 and 1969, Dr. Sacks and some of his colleagues made a major change at Mount Carmel by bringing the majority of their PE patients together into a single, organic, and self-governing community. This was done to give their patients a sense of belonging, instead of being treated as condemned prisoners in a vast and hopeless institution. The aim here was to improve their overall condition by establishing certain sympathies and kinships, and by relaxing the rigid staff/patient relationship.

Some of the patients introduced in this story are: Leonard, Rose, Hester, Rolando, and Miriam. Most of the patients no longer had visitors but Leonard's mother, Mrs. L., visited every day to take care of her son. Some of these patients were still able to walk freely using two sticks and they spoke well enough to be understood by the staff. On the other hand, another subset of these patients were less ambulatory —they were unable even to turn over in their beds, or just sat motionless in their wheelchairs for hours.

Notes

1 **neurologist**「神経学者、神経科医」　4 **trance-like state**「昏睡（昏迷）状態」　7 **nervous system**「神経系」　9 **afflict**「(精神的・肉体的に) 苦しめる、悩ます」　10- **post-encephalitic syndrome**「脳炎後症候群」　11 **a collection of neurological and psychiatric disorders**「神経・精神障害の集積」　12 **parkinsonism** ①「パーキンソン病、振せん麻痺」(**Parkinson's disease; shaking palsy; trembling palsy**) 脳のドパミン産生細胞の低下によって起こるとされている神経疾患。指や手の震え、筋肉の硬直、小きざみ歩行、前傾姿勢、仮面状顔貌その他の症状が見られる。②「パーキンソン症候群」パーキンソン病に類似した脳筋肉の硬直による脳の病気一般をさす。この文章では②の意で使われている。　13 **variable**「変わりやすい、定まらない」　13 **course and pattern**「進行と傾向」　14 **post-encephalitic patient**「脳炎後遺症患者」　17 **comprise**「～より成る」　24 **a single, organic, and self-governing community**「一つの組織的な自治コミュニティー」　26 **condemned prisoner**「有罪の判決を受けた囚人」　26 **vast**「広大な」　28 **rigid**「硬直した」　35 **subset**「一団」　35 **ambulatory**「歩行できる、床に就ききりでない」

True or False Questions

1. (　) Most of the encephalitis lethargica patients died in the 1920's.
2. (　) At Mount Carmel Hospital in 1969, the staff and post-encephalitic (PE) patients had a close relationship.
3. (　) When Dr. Sacks joined Mount Carmel, there was unanimous support, among hospital staff, for his ideas.
4. (　) Many PE patients were found throughout the world in the 1960s.
5. (　) Mrs. L. always visited Leonard.

Ⅳ USEFUL EXPRESSIONS

The following sentences were used in Dr. Sacks' original book. Use the hints below to help you to accurately translate the sentences into Japanese.

次の英文は、すべてサックス博士の小説 ***Awakenings*** に出てくるものです。それぞれの語（句）の注を参考に、日本語に訳してみましょう。

1. L-dopa was considered an <u>experimental drug</u> at this time, and I needed to get (from <u>the Food and Drug Administration</u>) a special investigator's license to use it.

   experimental drug「実験段階の薬、実験的薬剤」 **(the) Food and Drug Administration**「米国食品医薬品局」厚生省の一局で、食料品、医薬品、化粧品の検査や取り締まり、認可などを行う。略 **FDA**。

2. It was a <u>condition of</u> such licenses that one use <u>'orthodox' methods</u>, including a <u>double-blind trial</u>, <u>coupled with</u> presentation of results in <u>quantitative form</u>.

   condition of ～「～の条件」 **'orthodox' method(s)**「一般的（正統的）な方法」 **double-blind trial**「二重盲検試験」結果が出るまで、治療条件や患者分類を伏せておく臨床試験。 **coupled with**「～と相まった」 **quantitative form**「計量的形態、計量値」

3. In the winter of 1916-17, in <u>Vienna</u> and other cities, a 'new' illness suddenly appeared, and <u>rapidly spread</u>, over the next three years, to <u>become worldwide in its distribution</u>.

Vienna「ウィーン」 **rapidly spread**「急速に広まる」 **become world-wide in its distribution**「世界中にその分布を広める」

4. Mount Carmel was opened shortly after <u>the First World War</u> for <u>war-veterans</u> with injuries of the nervous system, and for the expected <u>victims of the sleeping-sickness</u>.

___

___

(the) First World War「第一次世界大戦」 **war-veteran(s)**「復員兵」 **victim(s) of the sleeping-sickness**「眠り病（(嗜眠性脳炎）の患者）」

5. At Mount Carmel, nurses, <u>aides</u>, <u>orderlies</u>, <u>physiotherapists</u>, <u>occupational therapists</u> and <u>speech therapists</u> gave themselves <u>unstintingly</u> and with love to the patients.

___

___

aide(s)「介護補助者」 **orderly(ies)**「付き添い」 **physiotherapist(s) (physical therapist)**「理学療法士」 **occupational therapist(s)**「作業療法士」 **speech therapist(s)**「言語聴覚士（言語療法士）」 **unstintingly**「惜しみなく、無条件で」

Ⅴ LISTENING FOCUS　　　　　　　　　　　　　　　　　CD 3

Please listen to Chapter 1-Dialog 1 and fill in the blanks with appropriate words, expressions, or phrases.

次の会話を聞いて、空欄の英語を聞き取ってみましょう。

Dialog 1

Interviewer: Can you please tell us what changes you have made at Mount Carmel?
Dr. Sacks: Well, when I arrived there in 1966, almost half of the post-encephalitic patients were in a state of pathological sleep. We knew we had to improve their quality of life.
Interviewer: (　　　)(　　　)(　　　)(　　　)(　　　)?
Dr. Sacks: Well, first of all, we had to bring all of the patients into one unit to make a self-governing community. We searched for lost relatives and I tried to (　　　)(　　　)(　　　) the (　　　) (　　　).
Interviewer: Were you successful?

Dr. Sacks: (　　　), (　　　) (　　　) (　　　) (　　　) (　　　). There was some establishment of sympathies and kinships and a thawing in the staff/patient divisions.
Interviewer: And the patients?
Dr. Sacks: After such a long time and considering the severity of the illness, some patients who awoke exhibited a kind of serenity, which may have masked a feeling of hopelessness, whereas others had a clear sense of outrage (　　　) (　　　) (　　　) (　　　) (　　　).

VI MORE ABOUT AMERICAN HEALTH ISSUES

精神病医療の歴史

Psychiatric Institutions: mental hospitals, psychiatric hospitals（精神科病院）

　精神科病院とは、精神障害者の治療およびケアに必要な専門職員をもち、精神障害のある者の入院・外来設備を有する専門施設をいう。かつての精神病院は精神障害者を隔離、監禁することに主眼が置かれたが、現在は、薬物療法、精神療法、作業療法などをできるだけ開放した環境の中で行う治療とケアを目的としている。

　18世紀末から19世紀はじめのフランスで、ピネルが精神障害者を鎖から開放し、病院の閉鎖病棟の改善を図った。同じく19世紀のイギリスで、テュークがヨーク療養所を設立し、コノリーによる無拘束運動が広まったが、その処遇はまだまだ不当なものであった。1900年頃からようやくその研究がなされ、現代の精神医学の基礎が築かれた。しかしながら、世界大戦時に精神障害者は再び迫害を受けることとなった。第二次世界大戦後には、人間性の尊重が再認識され、精神病院の開放化が進められるようになり、本格的な治療体制へ移行されてきた。この作品の舞台となっている1960年代に、アメリカではようやく閉鎖的ケアから治療的ケアに移行し始めた。しかし、現在でも解決すべき問題点が多いのが現実である。

　日本では、1879年に上野に、東京府癲狂院が開設された。これが東京府巣鴨病院となり、1919年に巣鴨から世田谷へ移転され、東京府松沢病院となった。現在の世田谷区松沢にある東京都立松沢病院が、1973年の精神医学総合研究所の併設に伴って、名実共に日本の精神科の診療と研究の中心となっている。わが国の現状もまた、医療費や福祉費の問題を含め、考慮すべき問題は多い。

Ⅶ YOUR OPINIONS

次の英語の質問に対し、英語または日本語で答えてみましょう。さらにグループで話し合ってみるのもよいでしょう。

Q. Have you had any experiences with people who have suffered similar post-encephalitic syndromes or with people with general mental illness? Were these people friends, family members, or strangers? Would you like to share your experiences and knowledge with your group members?

_____

_____

_____

_____

Chapter 2

Life at Mount Carmel (2)

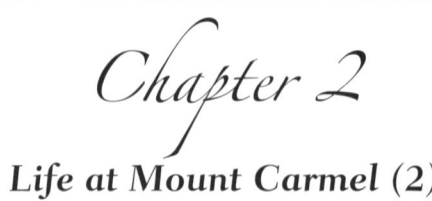

　患者の診察に従事している最中、サックス医師は丁度その時期にパーキンソン病の新薬として開発された薬に注目します。2年の考慮期間を経て、いよいよこの薬が患者達に投与されることになります。その結果は…

I PRE-READING

Bronx について

Mount Carmel Hospital is located in the Bronx, New York. How much do you know about the Bronx?

Fact 1: The Bronx is one of the five boroughs of New York City.
Fact 2: The borough is commonly called 'The Bronx,' but the official county name is just the 'Bronx', without the definite article 'The'.
Fact 3: The Bronx has a number of major attractions, including:
- Yankee Stadium, the home of the New York Yankees baseball club.
- The Bronx Zoo, which is the largest metropolitan zoo in the United States. It is home to over 4,000 animals, many of which are endangered or threatened species.
- The New York Botanical Garden, which was founded in 1891.

Fact 4: Although the Bronx has often been portrayed in popular culture as being a crime-ridden neighborhood of New York, the Bronx's crime rate has fluctuated over time and in recent years, the area has become relatively safe. Only certain parts of the borough are still typical of the poor urban areas of New York City.

II VOCABULARY & IDIOMATIC EXPRESSIONS

The following terms are used in the story below. Match each of the following words or phrases (①−⑥) with the correct definitions (meaning 'in context') from the box below (a−f). Also choose the appropriate Japanese translation (ア−カ) for each term.

　下の語（句）は、すべて **STORY** に出てくるものです。それぞれの英語の説明として、ふさわしいものを a～f の中から選びなさい。さらにその日本語の意味として、最もふさわしいものをア～カの中から選びなさい。

① administer　　　　　(　)(　)　②give way to　(　)(　)
③ throw oneself into (　)(　)　④syndrome　　(　)(　)
⑤ dose　　　　　　　　(　)(　)　⑥therapeutic　(　)(　)

> a) relating to the treatment or cure of a disease
> b) to eagerly start doing an activity using a lot of time and effort
> c) a measured amount of medicine
> d) to give someone medicine or drugs in a medical context
> e) a set of physical or mental problems that together signify a disease
> f) to change from the original state to a different state

ア　治療（法）の、治癒効果のある　　イ　（１回分の薬の）服用量、（薬の）一服
ウ　（〜に）移行する　　　　　　　　エ　（薬など）を投与する
オ　症候群　　　　　　　　　　　　　カ　（仕事などに）打ち込む

III COMPREHENSION

The following story will help you to understand life at Mount Carmel. Please read the story first and then answer the true or false questions below.

次の英文を読んで、正しいものにはT、間違っているものにはFをつけましょう。

STORY

　　Early in 1967, Dr. Cotzias and his colleagues published their report on the therapeutic success of their treatment of parkinsonism by administering massive doses of L-dopa, a drug which was only used experimentally at that time. Dr. Sacks read this report but hesitated to use it on his own post-encephalitic (PE) patients, mainly because their pathophysiological syndromes were much more complex and their situations were more difficult than those seen in Dr. Cotzias's patients. Furthermore, the cost of L-dopa was prohibitively high in 1967 or 1968, placing the drug beyond the reach of Mount Carmel Hospital, which was not a charity hospital and which was not attached to any university or foundation.

　　However, circumstances changed and in 1969, Dr. Sacks finally decided to administer L-dopa to his PE patients. In 1968, the Bronx endured a very hot summer, and because of this some of the PE patients got worse and died. This convinced Dr. Sacks that some drastic measures clearly needed to be taken. Moreover, towards the end of that year, the cost of L-dopa declined sharply. Finally, with great caution, Dr. Sacks began to treat the patients with L-dopa in March 1969. This was a revolutionary step as it had never before been tried on patients suffering from encephalitis lethargica.

At first, Dr. Sacks administered L-dopa only to Leonard. To everyone's surprise, Leonard finally woke up after thirty years. Encouraged by this initial success, Dr. Sacks threw himself into his work, giving L-dopa to the other PE patients. Most of the patients made remarkable progress and the treatment seemed to be a real miracle. Nevertheless, as the treatment outcomes became more complicated, the initial joy experienced by the patients, their families, and medical personnel, gave way to more subdued emotions.

Notes

2 **parkinsonism** ①「パーキンソン病、振せん麻痺」(**Parkinson's disease; shaking palsy; trembling palsy**) 脳のドーパミン産生細胞の低下によって起こるとされている神経疾患。指や手の震え、筋肉の硬直、小きざみ歩行、前傾姿勢、仮面状顔貌その他の症状が見られる。②「パーキンソン症候群」パーキンソン病に類似した症状を示す、流行性脳炎や梅毒などで錐体外路系が冒される疾患。この文章では①の意で使われている。 3 **massive dose of ~**「大量の～」 4 **experimentally**「実験的に」 6 **patho-physiological**「病態生理学的な」病態生理学とは、病気でみられる機能の乱れ、すなわち構造上の欠陥と区別される機能上の変化を扱う。 8 **prohibitively high**「非常に高い」 10 **charity hospital**「慈善病院」 11 **foundation**「財団、社会事業団、協会」 15 **convince**「確信させる、納得させる」 15 **drastic measure**「思い切った処置、抜本策」 19 **revolutionary step**「画期的な進歩」 24 **remarkable progress**「注目すべき進展」 27 **medical personnel**「医療関係者」 28 **subdued emotion**「沈んだ感情」

True or False Questions

1. (　) Immediately after learning of the success of the L-dopa treatment reported by Dr. Cotzias, Dr. Sacks was really happy and decided to use L-dopa on his patients.
2. (　) Dr. Sacks decided to give L-dopa to his PE patients because the drug worked so well on other PE patients.
3. (　) In 1969, Leonard was the only person to be administered L-dopa by Dr. Sacks at the Mount Carmel Hospital.
4. (　) The fierce summer heat in 1968 dramatically worsened the conditions of some PE patients.
5. (　) Mt. Carmel Hospital was able to purchase L-dopa in 1967.

IV USEFUL EXPRESSIONS

The following sentences were used in Dr. Sacks' original book. Use the hints below to help you to accurately translate the sentences into Japanese.

次の英文は、すべてサックス博士の小説 ***Awakenings*** に出てくるものです。それぞれの語（句）の注を参考に、日本語に訳してみましょう。

1. L-dopa is a 'miracle drug'—the term is used everywhere.

   _____

   _____

   'miracle drug'「奇跡の薬」

2. In 1920, the Vogts suggested that a specific treatment for parkinsonism, and related disorders, might become possible if this hypothetical chemical substance could be identified and administered.

   _____

   _____

   the Vogts「フォークト父子（親子）」　**hypothetical chemical substance**「仮説に基づいた化学物質」　**be identified and administered**「〜が明らかにされ、（患者に）投与される」

3. Both Leonard and his mother expressed uncertainty and ambivalence about the use of L-dopa; both of them had read about it, but neither had actually seen its effects.

   _____

   _____

   uncertainty「確信のなさ、疑念」　**ambivalence**「躊躇、ためらい」

4. They yearned incessantly for a twofold miracle—not only a cure for their sickness, but an indemnification for the loss of their lives.

   _____

   _____

   incessantly「絶え間なく」　**indemnification for**「〜の補償」

5. In the summer of 1970, then, in a letter to the Journal of the American Medical Association (JAMA), I reported these findings, describing the total effects of L-DOPA in 60 patients whom I had maintained on it for a year.

Journal of the American Medical Association (JAMA)「米国医師会雑誌（米国医師会によって刊行される、国際的な医学雑誌）」　**finding(s)**「答申、結果」

Ⅴ LISTENING FOCUS　　　　　　　　　　　　　　　CD 5

Please listen to Chapter 2-Dialog 2 and fill in the blanks with appropriate words, expressions, or phrases.

次の会話を聞いて、空欄の英語を聞き取ってみましょう。

Dialog 2

Leonard: We have to have a tour of all the United States so that I can tell people the Gospel of Life according to L-dopa.
Dr. Sacks: (　　　) (　　　) (　　　) (　　　) (　　　), Leonard?
Leonard: I've written the newspapers, congressmen and even the White House about L-dopa. Also, I don't understand why the nurses don't like me anymore.
Dr. Sacks: Leonard, (　　　) (　　　) (　　　) (　　　) (　　　) your yearnings have become more aggressive. The nurses' good humor has disappeared.
Leonard: I'm not weak and mild anymore. I'm a powerful king with artistic and sexual omnipotence.
Dr. Sacks: That is the drug talking.
Leonard: No, L-dopa is the power. L-dopa has given me the power that I have craved. I (　　　) (　　　) (　　　) (　　　) (　　　) for (　　　) (　　　).

VI MORE ABOUT AMERICAN HEALTH ISSUES

嗜眠性脳炎とは

Encephalitis lethargica

　流行性脳炎の一種。高熱と複雑な脳神経症状が見られ、著しい嗜眠傾向がある。症状としては、頭痛、睡眠障害、不随意運動、筋硬直などがある。急性期は通常4週間程度であるといわれる。死亡率は20%と高率で、予後は不良である。生存者には後遺症として高率にパーキンソン病の症状が出ることがあり、このためパーキンソン症候群の治療法がとられている。1916～1917年にウイーンで報告されたのをはじめに、1925年ごろまで世界各地で見られた。1940年以降の発生報告はほとんどない。病原体はウイルスと推定されているが、発生時にはウイルスを確認する適当な方法がなかったため、ついにその確認はされていない。

VII YOUR OPINIONS

次の英語の質問に対し、英語または日本語で答えてみましょう。さらに、グループで話し合ってみるのもよいでしょう。

Q1. What do you think of Dr. Sacks' initial hesitation in using L-dopa for his PE patients?

Q2. What would you do if you, as someone with a medical or a paramedical background, were to find yourself in a similar position, today, to that faced by Dr. Sacks in 1967?

Awakenings

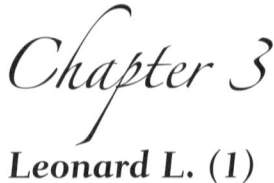
Leonard L. (1)

　サックス医師が最初にL-dopaを投与したのはレナードでした。どうして彼はレナードを選んだのでしょう。サックス医師とレナードとの出会いはどのようなものだったのでしょうか。

I PRE-READING
Experimental Drugs（実験段階の薬の使用）
How much do you know about experimental drugs ? Decide if the statements below are T (True) or F (False).

1. It takes about one year for an experimental drug to receive government approval in the US. （　）
2. To receive approval, the experimental drug must be clinically tested on humans. （　）
3. After being approved, the experimental drug, in most cases, is usually easily obtained at most US pharmacies. （　）
4. When an experimental drug is not approved, we can only conclude that the drug must be ineffective. （　）
5. Drugs which aren't approved in the first application are sometimes approved in subsequent attempts. （　）

II VOCABULARY & IDIOMATIC EXPRESSIONS
The following terms are used in the story below. Match each of the following words or phrases (①-⑥) with the correct definitions (meaning 'in context') from the box below (a-f). Also choose the appropriate Japanese translation (ア-カ) for each term.

下の語（句）は，すべて **STORY** に出てくるものです。それぞれの英語の説明として、ふさわしいものをa～fの中から選びなさい。さらにその日本語の意味として、最もふさわしいものをア～カの中から選びなさい。

① be petrified　　　　　　　　（　）（　）　② chronological age　（　）（　）
③ be admitted to（hospital）（　）（　）　④ resentful　　　　　　（　）（　）
⑤ dystrophic change　　　　（　）（　）　⑥ introspective　　　　（　）（　）

a) the number of years a person has lived as opposed to their level of physical, mental, or emotional development
b) unable to move, frozen
c) serious physical change due to a illness in which the muscles become weaker over a period of time
d) tending to think deeply about one's own thoughts, feelings etc.
e) to formally accept as a patient
f) feeling of anger because something has happened that one thinks is unfair

ア　生活年齢、暦年齢　　　　　　　イ　憤慨している、怒っている
ウ　（身体が）カチカチに硬くなる、硬直化する
エ　ジストロフィーによって起こる（筋力が弱まるなどの）身体的な変化
オ　内省の、内省的な　　　　　　　カ　入院する

III COMPREHENSION

The story below will help you to understand Dr. Sacks' patient, Leonard. Please read the passage and then answer the true or false questions that follow.

次の英文を読んで、正しいものにはT、間違っているものにはFをつけましょう。

STORY

Dr. Sacks first met Leonard in the spring of 1966. At that time, Leonard was forty-six, completely speechless, and without voluntary motion except for minute movements of the right hand. He seemed a good deal younger than his chronological age. He showed extreme rigidity of the neck, trunk, and limbs, and marked dystrophic changes in his hands, which were no larger than those of a child. Leonard experienced the first post-encephalitic (PE) symptoms at age fifteen, when his right hand started to become stiff, weak, pale and shrunken. With his small hands, Leonard could tap out text on a spelling-board, and this slow, painful process had been his only mode of communication, until he was given L-dopa in 1969.

Soon after his first PE symptoms, there was a gradual spread and progression of Leonard's disability. Despite this, Leonard was able to graduate with honors from Harvard University. In fact, he was able to continue post-graduate studies and had actually come close to completing a thesis for his PhD at age twenty-seven, at which point the severity of his disease brought his studies to a total halt. Leonard then spent the next three years at home and was admitted to the Mount Carmel Hospital at age thirty, when he was almost totally petrified.

There was a complex relationship between Leonard and his mother, Mrs. L.. Mrs. L. visited her son frequently and took care of him for ten hours on each visit. While she clearly derived some pleasure from her mothering role, she also resented the way in which her life was being 'sacrificed' to care for Leonard. Leonard had, in effect, become a 'parasite.' For his part, although Leonard expressed some sense of joy at his mother's attention, he was also resentful of his almost total dependence on her.

In spite of his extremely dependent and immobile state, Leonard was intelligent, cultivated, sophisticated, and an avid reader. In fact, his disability did not prevent him from continuing his intellectual pursuits— he had managed to actually become the librarian at the hospital and also produced monthly book reviews in the hospital magazine. Dr. Sacks was very impressed with Leonard's introspective and investigative passion, which exceeded that of almost any other of Dr. Sack's patients. Dr. Sacks regarded Leonard as an 'ideal' patient due to a special combination— Leonard's disease was in a highly progressed state and yet he maintained an intense investigative intelligence. This unique situation allowed Dr. Sacks to learn more about parkinsonism, PE illness, suffering, and human nature, than anything from the rest of his patients combined.

Notes

2 **speechless**「言葉をしゃべれない、口が利けない」 2-**voluntary motion**「随意運動」 3 **minute movement**「わずかな動き」 5 **trunk**「人や動物の胴体」 5 **limb**「(頭部・胴体と区別して) 肢：手、腕、足」 8 **stiff**「硬い、硬直した」 8 **pale**「血の気のない、青白い」 8 **shrunken**「縮んだ」 9 **spelling-board**「文字盤、スペル盤」 14 **graduate with honors from** ～「(大学など) を優等で卒業する」 15 **post-graduate**「大学院の」 17 **bring** ～ **to a total halt**「～を完全に中止させる」 22 **derive**「見出す、得る」 23 **resent**「腹を立てる」 24 '**parasite**'「厄介者」 28 **cultivated**「教養のある」 28 **avid reader**「熱心な読書家」 29 **intellectual pursuit**「知的な探求」 30 **librarian**「図書館員、司書」 35 **highly progressed state**「かなり進展した病状」 36 **intense investigative intelligence**「熱心な探求的知性」

True or False Questions

1. (　) Leonard was a very smart person who loved to read books.
2. (　) After Leonard was admitted to Mount Carmel, he could not read books at all.

3. (　) Leonard and his mother had a very complicated relationship.
4. (　) Leonard looked older than he really was.
5. (　) Dr. Sacks learned a great deal from Leonard.

IV USEFUL EXPRESSIONS

The following sentences were used in Dr. Sacks' original book. Use the hints below to help you to accurately translate the sentences into Japanese.

次の英文は、すべてサックス博士の小説 ***Awakenings*** に出てくるものです。それぞれの語（句）の注を参考に、日本語に訳してみましょう。

1. He suffered from frequent 'micro-crises'—upturnings of the eyeballs, associated with transient inability to move or respond.

   _____

   _____

   suffer from ～「～を被る、～に苦しめられる」　**'micro-crisis'**「ミクロ発作」
   upturning(s)「上を向くこと」　**associated with** ～「～と関係した」
   transient「一時的な、一過性の」

2. Leonard was indeed continually buried in books, and had few or no friends.

   _____

   _____

   be buried in ～「～に埋もれている」

3. On his admission he was at once given charge of the hospital library.

   _____

   _____

   be given charge of ～「～の管理を任せられる」

4. He could do little but read, and he did nothing but read.

   _____

   _____

   do little but ～「～以外はほとんどしない」　**do nothing but** ～「～ばかりする」

5. "What's it like being the way you are? What would you compare it to?" He spelt out the following answer: "Caged. Deprived. Like Rilke's 'Panther'."

_____

_____

   Rilke's 'Panther'「リルケ（フランスの詩人）の『豹』」

6. There existed an <u>intense and mutual dependence</u> between Leonard and his mother.

_____

_____

   intense and mutual dependence「極度の相互依存関係」

V LISTENING FOCUS　　　　　　　　　　　　　CD 7

Please listen to Chapter 3-Dialog 3 and fill in the blanks with appropriate words, expressions, or phrases.

次の会話を聞いて、空欄の英語を聞き取ってみましょう。

Dialog 3 （レナードが文字盤によってサックス博士とかわした会話）

Leonard:　This is a human zoo.
Dr. Sacks: (　　　)(　　　)(　　　)(　　　)(　　　)(　　　)?
Leonard:　Look around. Everyone in this ward is caged. Deprived. Just like animals.
Dr. Sacks: (　　　)(　　　)(　　　)(　　　)?
Leonard:　I feel meek.
Dr. Sacks: (　　　)(　　　)(　　　)(　　　)(　　　)?
Leonard:　No.
Dr. Sacks: (　　　)(　　　)
Leonard:　Most of the time I feel meek, but other times I feel great power and violence locked up in me. I'm trapped in myself.
Dr. Sacks: Trapped?
Leonard:　I have no exit. This stupid body is a prison with windows but no doors.
Dr. Sacks: (　　　)(　　　)(　　　)(　　　)?
Leonard:　I am what I am. I am part of the world. My disease and deformity are part of the world. They are beautiful in a way like a dwarf or a toad.

VI MORE ABOUT AMERICAN HEALTH ISSUES

パーキンソン病とパーキンソン症候群－症状とその治療方法

Parkinson's disease（パーキンソン病）

　英国の医師ジェームズ・パーキンソンが1817年に初めて報告した病気。彼の名をとって、パーキンソン病と呼ばれるようになった。ドーパミンの著しい減少により脳の変性をきたす疾患で、筋硬直、全身の動作減少、手指の震顫、姿勢保持困難などを主な症状として呈する。治療にはL-ドーパやドーパミンの放出を促すアマンタジンなどの服用や抗コリン薬などの薬物用法などが行われている。難病に指定されている。

parkinsonism, parkinsonian syndrome（パーキンソン症候群）

　パーキンソン症候群は、パーキンソン病と似た症状を示す疾患で、その原因として特発性のいわゆるパーキンソン病ではなく、脳血管障害や薬物、流行性脳炎、梅毒、一酸化炭素中毒などによって錐体外路系が冒された場合に起こる。

VII YOUR OPINIONS

次の英語の質問に対し、英語または日本語で答えてみましょう。さらにグループで話し合ってみるのもよいでしょう。

Q1. What do you think is the most striking aspect of Leonard's personality? Consider his activities in the context of his disability.

Q2. Why do you think Dr. Sacks chose Leonard as the first patient to receive L-dopa?

Chapter 4
Leonard L. (2)

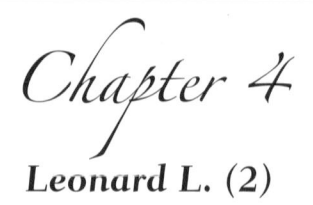

いよいよレナードに L-dopa が投与されます。最初の反応はどういうものだったのでしょう。30 年の空白を経て目覚めたレナードは現実社会にどのように対処するのでしょうか。

I PRE-READING

L-dopa（L-ドーパの効用と副作用）

All types of medication have both positive and negative effects. Some of the improvements and side effects brought on by the L-dopa treatment are listed below. Please characterize each of the following symptoms (excerpted and paraphrased from the story below) as either a positive (P) or a negative (N) effect.

(1) vanishing sense of hostility, anxiety, and tensions (   )
(2) feeling a sense of harmony and safety (   )
(3) determined to rid the 'polluted' world of its evils (   )
(4) feeling insatiable passions and greeds (   )

II VOCABULARY & IDIOMATIC EXPRESSIONS

The following terms are used in the story below. Match each of the following words or phrases (①-⑥) with the correct definitions (meaning 'in context') from the box below (a-f). Also choose the appropriate Japanese translation (ア-カ) for each term.

下の語（句）は、すべて **STORY** に出てくるものです。それぞれの英語の説明として、ふさわしいものを a～f の中から選びなさい。さらにその日本語の意味として、最もふさわしいものをア～カの中から選びなさい。

① assessment   (   ) (   )   ② appreciate   (   ) (   )
③ autobiography (   ) (   )   ④ be empowered (   ) (   )
⑤ innumerable   (   ) (   )   ⑥ be destined for (   ) (   )

a) be certain about achieving a particular fate
b) recognize the full worth of
c) an account of a person's life written by that person
d) be authorized and enabled to do something
e) a judgment about a person or situation after careful consideration
f) very many or too many to be counted

ア 〈人が〉(…を受ける) 運命にある　　イ 自伝
ウ 能力を与えられる、権力を与えられる　エ 味わう、真価を認める
オ (事態に対する) 判定、評価、所見　　カ 非常に多くの、数え切れない

III COMPREHENSION

The story below will help you to understand Dr. Sacks' patient, Leonard. Please read and answer the true or false questions below.

次の英文を読んで、正しいものにはT、間違っているものにはFをつけましょう。

STORY

Leonard received his first L-dopa in early March 1969, after which the dose was raised by degrees. It took two weeks for any major effects to be seen, at which time Leonard experienced a sudden 'conversion' as the rigidity vanished from all his limbs and he felt energized and empowered. He was now able to do things that had not been possible since his twenty-fifth year—to write and type, to rise from his chair, to walk with some assistance, and to speak loudly and clearly. By the end of March, Leonard enjoyed a strong sense of mobility, health, and happiness which he had last experienced thirty years before. Leonard seemed intoxicated with appreciating the beauty of everything around him, and began living life to the fullest.

Leonard was determined to experience everything in his new world. He said, "I have been hungry and yearning all my life, and now I am full. I want nothing more." This seemed consistent with Dr. Sacks' own assessment—he noted a vanishing of hostility, anxiety, and tensions in Leonard.

Unfortunately, this miracle didn't last long. In April, hints of trouble appeared. Leonard's sense of harmony and ease was replaced by a pathological sense of 'purpose.' He felt destined for a specific mission and fate—he saw himself as a Messiah, or the Son of God, sent to rid the 'polluted' world of innumerable 'devils.' Moreover, whereas Leonard had previously felt satisfied, he now experienced insatiable sexual yearnings and other passions.

At the start of June, Leonard finally decided to try to regain control by working on an autobiography, which he hoped would 'cast out the devils.' Initially, this seemed to work and Leonard decided that he needed absolute solitude and concentration. He therefore pushed his mother to take a vacation, saying that he did not need her so much now. This greatly upset Mrs. L. and it now became apparent that she, in fact, depended on Leonard—she needed to take care of him. Indeed, Mrs. L. blamed the L-dopa treatment for 'taking Leonard away from her.'

Notes

2 **major effect**「主な効果、影響」 3 **'conversion'**「転換、変化」 8 **mobility**「可動性、運動性」 9 **intoxicated**「興奮した、うっとりした」 19 **pathological sense of 'purpose'**「病的な意向」 19 **mission**「使命」 20 **Messiah**「救世主」 20 **Son of God**「神の子」 22 **insatiable**「飽くことを知らない、貪欲な」 25 **-'cast out the devils'**「悪魔を追い払う」 27 **absolute solitude**「絶対的な孤独」 29 **become apparent**「明らかになる」

True or False Questions

1. (　) Because Leonard wanted to concentrate on the writing of his autobiography, he told his mother to take a vacation.
2. (　) L-dopa started to work for Leonard immediately after it was first administered to him.
3. (　) The L-dopa treatment allowed Leonard to recover many of his physical qualities.
4. (　) Leonard showed a significant change in his mind-set in April 1969.
5. (　) Mrs. L was really happy with how focused Leonard was on his autobiography.

IV USEFUL EXPRESSIONS

The following sentences were used in Dr. Sacks' original book. Use the hints below to help you to accurately translate the sentences into Japanese.

次の英文は、すべてサックス博士の小説 ***Awakenings*** に出てくるものです。それぞれの語（句）の注を参考に、日本語に訳してみましょう。

1. "…I feel like a man in love. I have broken through the barriers which <u>cut me off from</u> love."

   _____

   _____

   cut ~ off from…「～を…から遮断する」

2. "L-dopa is a blessed drug, it has given me back the possibility of life. It has <u>opened me out</u> where I <u>was clammed tight-shut</u> before."

   _____

   _____

   open ~ out「～を解き放つ」　　**be clammed tight-shut**「硬く閉ざされる」

3. Tics appeared at this time, and <u>grew more numerous daily</u>: <u>sudden impulses</u> and <u>tics</u> of the eyes, <u>grimaces</u>, <u>cluckings</u>, and <u>lightning-quick scratchings</u>.

   _____

   _____

   grow more numerous daily「毎日その数が増えてく」　　**sudden impulse(s)**「突然の衝動」　　**tic(s)**「チック」特に顔面・肩・首などの急激な痙攣（けいれん）性で無痛の不随意筋収縮　　**grimace(s)**「顔のひきつり、しかみ」　　**clucking(s)**「舌打ち」　　**lightning-quick scratching(s)**「矢のように早く（皮膚を）かきむしること」

4. He typed almost <u>ceaselessly</u>—twelve to fifteen hours a day, and when he typed he indeed '<u>came together</u>,' and found himself free from his tics and <u>distractions</u>.

   _____

   _____

   ceaselessly「絶え間なく」　　**'come together'**「統一する」　　**distraction(s)**「気を散らすこと」

5. "…. He has <u>pushed me away</u>. He only <u>thinks of himself</u>. <u>I need to be needed</u>—it's the main need I have. Len's been <u>my baby</u> for the last thirty years, and you've <u>taken him away</u> with your <u>darned</u> EL-Dopey!"

   _____

push ~ away「~を押しやる」 think of oneself「自分だけのことしか考えない」
S need to be needed「S は必要とされたい」 one's baby「~のかわいい子供（息子）」 take ~ away「~を奪い去る」 darned「とんでもない」

V LISTENING FOCUS　　　　　　　　　　　　　　　　　CD 9

Please listen to Chapter 4-Dialog 4 and fill in the blanks with appropriate words, expressions, or phrases.

次の会話を聞いて、空欄の英語を聞き取ってみましょう。

Dialog 4

Leonard: The city at night is like a jewel.
Dr. Sacks: (　　　)(　　　)(　　　)(　　　)(　　　)(　　　)?
Leonard: (　　　)(　　　)(　　　) a (　　　)(　　　)(　　　). It is what I have been yearning for all my life.
Dr. Sacks: Leonard, I'm really happy that (　　　)(　　　)(　　　)(　　　)(　　　)(　　　).
Leonard: Yes, the sense of friendship and kinship I feel now is even better than what I experienced before the parkinsonism. *For this* (　　　)(　　　)(　　　)(　　　), my life of disease. Everyone should feel as good as I do now.

VI MORE ABOUT AMERICAN HEALTH ISSUES

> 実験段階の薬と治験
>
> **Experimental Drugs**
>
> 　実験段階の薬（実験的薬剤）とは、まだ認可を受けていない薬、その実験段階にある薬のことをいう。薬を販売するには、アメリカでは、「(米国)食品医薬品局（the Food and Drug Administration 略 FDA）」という厚生省の一局が、食料品、医薬品、化粧品の検査や取り締まり、認可などを行う。日本の場合、厚生労働省の認可が必要になる。いずれの場合も、厚生労働省からの認可を得るためには、安全性、有効性などを適正な基準に沿って行われる試験、つまり治験を通過しなければならない。Chapter 12, 13 (Pre-reading) でアメリカの治験（臨床試験）についての説明があるので、治験や、新薬の認可が下りる過程を日米の違いなどから、さらに考えてみよう。

Ⅶ YOUR OPINIONS

次の英語の質問に対し、英語または日本語で答えてみましょう。さらにグループで話し合ってみるのもよいでしょう。

Q. How would you characterize the relationship between Leonard and his mother?

Ⅷ MEDICAL ENGLISH ENHANCER（英語で調べてみよう）

Complete a short (5-6 sentences) summary of the following medical term(s). Use English references as your source material.

"codependence"（共依存）または "interdependence"（相互依存）ついて英語の文献で調べ、それを5行程度の英文でまとめてみましょう。そして、レナードと彼の母親の関係を考えてみましょう。

_____

_____

_____

_____

_____

Chapter 5
Leonard L. (3)

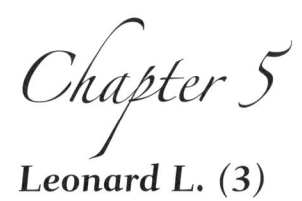

　レナードは薬の副作用と闘い続けます。果たしてサックス医師は、レナードにもう一度目覚めを取り戻させることができるのでしょうか。

I PRE-READING
Amantadine（アマンタジンの効用と副作用）
Have you ever heard of amantadine?

Fact 1: Amantadine is an antiviral medication used to prevent or treat certain types of influenza.
Fact 2: Amantadine is also given as an adjunct for the treatment of Parkinson's disease, where it is used either as monotherapy, or together with L-dopa.
Fact 3: Amantadine has been used with L-dopa to treat L-dopa-related motor fluctuations and L-dopa-related dyskinesias.
Fact 4: Amantadine has significant anti-cholinergic activity and this may explain the central nervous system (CNS) side-effects often associated with this drug.
Fact 5: Some of the CNS side-effects include nervousness, anxiety, agitation, insomnia, and exacerbations of pre-existing seizure disorders and psychiatric symptoms in patients with schizophrenia or Parkinson's disease.

II VOCABULARY & IDIOMATIC EXPRESSIONS

The following terms are used in the story below. Match each of the following words or phrases (①−⑥) with the correct definitions (meaning 'in context') from the box below (a−f). Also choose the appropriate Japanese translation (ア−カ) for each term.

下の語（句）は、すべて **STORY** に出てくるものです。それぞれの英語の説明として、ふさわしいものをa〜fの中から選びなさい。さらにその日本語の意味として、最もふさわしいものをア〜カの中から選びなさい。

① hallucination　　　（　）（　）　② manifest　　　　（　）（　）
③ assimilate　　　　（　）（　）　④ tic　　　　　　　（　）（　）
⑤ therapeutic benefit（　）（　）　⑥ precaution　　　　（　）（　）

> a) a measure taken in advance to prevent something dangerous, unpleasant or inconvenient from happening
> b) become apparent or obvious through the appearance of feelings, attitudes, or features
> c) a sudden, uncontrolled movement of a muscle, often in the face
> d) to become part of or to understand and accept experiences, information, or ideas
> e) positive result of a course of treatment, medication, or behavior
> f) something you see, feel, hear, or experience that is not really there; usually caused by a drug or mental illness

ア　治療的効果　　イ　予防策　　ウ　同化、適合、順応させる
エ　幻覚　　　　　オ　明らかにする、証明する　　カ　チック

III COMPREHENSION

The story below will help you to understand Dr. Sacks' patient, Leonard. Please read and answer the true or false questions below.

次の英文を読んで、正しいものにはT、間違っているものにはFをつけましょう。

STORY — CD 10

By the end of June, and throughout July, Leonard was constantly violent and in such a frenzied state that special precautions were required. His sexual and hostile impulses began to take the form of hallucinations. Sudden haltings and blocks manifested in his speech, his writings, and even in his walking and movements. During this period, Leonard began showing episodes where he oscillated from an intensely excited state to one of severe exhaustion. At first, these switches seemed to be related to the time of L-dopa administration and, to some extent, were controllable. But later, such switches emerged without relationship to dosage times, and reducing his total intake of L-dopa had no effect at all on his oscillations. How and why these oscillations came about were never resolved.

When Leonard was finally restricted to a tiny room and deprived of his belongings, he spiraled into a suicidal depression. Dr. Sacks stopped the L-dopa treatment at the end of July and three days later, Leonard's tics and psychoses suddenly stopped. By August, Leonard had returned to his original motionless state.

In September 1969, Leonard requested the L-dopa treatment be restarted but although he had become extraordinarily sensitive to the drug (he now reacted to 50 mg/day versus the 5,000 mg/day he had originally required,) this time, there was only a pathological response without any therapeutic benefits. Leonard was clearly expecting this, as he indicated to Dr. Sacks, using his letter-board, "I told you so. You will never see anything like April again."

Soon after, Dr. Sacks gave Leonard amantadine, which has effects similar to, but milder than, those of L-dopa. The therapeutic benefits of this drug also diminished with time such that in March 1972, at his eleventh and final trial of amantadine, Leonard experienced only pathological effects. Leonard then said, "This is the end of the line. I have had it with drugs. There is no more you can do with me."

Leonard used his strength and intelligence to assimilate the tumultuous results from years of drug treatments. As Leonard himself put it, "It was wonderful, terrible, dramatic, and comic. It is finally—sad, and that's all there is to it."

Notes

2 **frenzied state**「錯乱した状態」 3 **impulse**「衝動」 4 **halting and block**「口ごもりや妨害」 6 **episode**「症状の出現」 6 **oscillate**「揺れる」 6-**intensely excited state**「激しく興奮した状態」 11 **oscillation**「振れ」 13 **be restricted to a tiny room**「小さな部屋に隔離される」 13 **be deprived of** ～「～を取り上げられる」 14 **spiral into** ～「らせん状に～へ落下する」 14 **suicidal depression**「自殺的なうつ状態」 16 **psychosis**「精神障害」 21 **pathological response**「病的反応」 24 **letter-board**「文字盤」 29 **pathological effect**「病的効果」 29 **end of the line**「最後、我慢できる限界」 30 **have it with**「～に別れを告げる」 32 **tumultuous**「混乱した、無秩序の」

True or False Questions

1. (　) Even though eventually L-dopa did not work for Leonard, amantadine which was similar to but weaker than L-dopa, did work.
2. (　) In spite of the unsuccessful course of treatments, Leonard was finally able to come to terms with the whole experience.
3. (　) Leonard was given amantadine a total of three times in eleven years.
4. (　) Leonard asked Dr. Sacks to re-start the L-dopa treatment even though he had had negative experiences on the L-dopa regimen.
5. (　) In September 1969, when Dr. Sacks began the L-dopa treatment, it was not effective so Leonard's dosage was increased.

IV USEFUL EXPRESSIONS

The following sentences were used in Dr. Sacks' original book. Use the hints below to help you to accurately translate the sentences into Japanese.

次の英文は、すべてサックス博士の小説 ***Awakenings*** に出てくるものです。それぞれの語（句）の注を参考に、日本語に訳してみましょう。

1. Leonard returned to his violently frenzied and fragmented state.

    one's violently frenzied and fragmented state「暴力的な錯乱と人格の崩壊した状態」

2. His psychoses and tics continued for another three days, of their own momentum, and then suddenly came to a stop.

    psychosis（**pl. psychoses**）「（重症の）精神障害」　**one's own momentum**「独自の勢い」

3. He 'opened up' again to me, tapping his thoughts on his original letter board.

    'open up'「心を開く」　**tap one's thoughts on ～**「～に自らの思いを打ち込む」

4. His reaction to this way was initially very favorable, though lacking the intensity of the effects of L-dopa.

    be initially very favorable「最初はとても良い」　**(the) intensity of the effect(s) of ～**「～の強い効き目」

5. With each <u>successive use of amantadine</u>, the therapeutic effects became less marked and shorter in <u>duration</u>, and the <u>pathological effects</u> more marked.

_____

_____

successive use of amantadine「アマンタジンの継続使用」　**duration**「持続時間」　**pathological effect(s)**「病的効果」

V LISTENING FOCUS　　　　　　　　　　　CD 11

Please listen to Chapter 5-Dialog 5 and fill in the blanks with appropriate words, expressions, or phrases.

次の会話を聞いて、空欄の英語を聞き取ってみましょう。

Dialog 5

In 1972, the effectiveness of the treatments was shorter in duration. Leonard became rather pessimistic and negative about the continued use of amantadine.

Leonard: This is the end of the line. I have had it with drugs. There is no more that you can do for me.
Dr. Sacks: (　　　)(　　　)(　　　)?
Leonard: At first, Dr. Sacks, I thought L-dopa was (　　　)(　　　)(　　　)(　　　) in (　　　)(　　　) and I blessed you for giving me "the Elixir of Life."
Dr. Sacks: But (　　　)(　　　)(　　　)(　　　)?
Leonard: Everything went bad. I thought it was the worst thing in the world, a deathly poison, a drug which sent one to the depths of hell, and I cursed you for giving it to me.
Dr. Sacks: So, (　　　)(　　　)(　　　)(　　　)?
Leonard: I'm best left alone—no more drugs. I've broken through barriers which I had all my life. And now, I'll stay myself, and you can keep your L-dopa.

VI MORE ABOUT AMERICAN HEALTH ISSUES

アメリカの病院－その歴史1　History of American Hospitals (part 1)

　アメリカの病院の発祥は、1600年代のイギリスの植民地時代に、それぞれの植民地で、貧窮者、孤児、高齢者や病人の救済施設として始まった。植民地での生活が安定するにつれ、その救済施設は病人を中心とする慈善施設となり、自治体病院へと発展していく。1700年代中期になると、寄付金を基に設立され運営されるボランタリー病院の建設が始まった。当時の自治体病院とボランタリー病院は、治療のための医療施設というよりは慈善施設としての役割が高く、衛生状態も決して良くはなかった。そのため、中流以上の人々は、医師に自宅まで往診してもらうことを好んだ。しかし南北戦争後、医療技術や医療機器の向上により、病院は医療施設としての役割を持つようになった。

VII YOUR OPINIONS

次の英語の質問に対し、英語または日本語で答えてみましょう。さらに、グループで話し合ってみるのもよいでしょう。

Q1. How would you respond to someone exhibiting the types of behavior Leonard showed with his 'Messiah complex' and with his other violent actions?

_____

_____

_____

_____

_____

_____

Q2. Do you think that the use of amantadine was advisable in this case?

_____

_____

_____

_____

Ⅷ MEDICAL ENGLISH ENHANCER（英語で調べてみよう）

Complete a short (5-6 sentences) summary of the following medical term(s). Use English references as your source material.

"Messiah complex"（メサイヤ・コンプレックス）について英語の文献で調べ、それを5行程度の英文でまとめてみましょう。それを参考にレナードにこれが起こった要因と可能と思われる対処策を考えてみましょう。

_____

_____

_____

_____

_____

Chapter 6
Rose R.

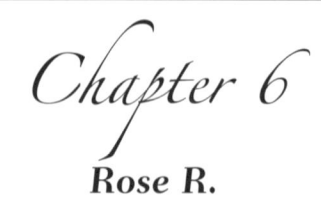

　ニューヨークの裕福な家に生まれ育ったローズは、21歳まで何不自由のない幸福な暮らしをしていました。しかしその年、嗜眠性脳炎を発症し、彼女の人生は一変しました。幸いにも家族の介護を受けていたローズでしたが、9年後にはマウント・カーメルに入院しなければならなくなりました。それから30年後、サックス医師は彼女を初めて診察し、やがて L-dopa を投与することにしますが…

I PRE-READING

Psychiatric Care Team-members（精神科病棟で働く人々）

Psychiatrists in many psychiatric wards often work cooperatively, with other healthcare professionals, to develop therapeutic treatments plans specifically customized to help individual patients regain their mental and physical health. Any combination of the following healthcare specialists may work at psychiatric wards.

Match each of the following terms（1－5）with the appropriate Japanese translation（ア－オ）.

1. speech therapist　　（　　　）　　2. occupational therapist　（　　　）
3. physical therapist　 （　　　）　　4. pharmacist　　　　　　（　　　）
5. music therapist　　 （　　　）

ア　薬剤師　　　　　イ　作業療法士　　　ウ　理学療法士
エ　言語聴覚士（言語療法士）　　　　　　オ　音楽療法士

II VOCABULARY & IDIOMATIC EXPRESSIONS

The following terms are used in the story below. Match each of the following words or phrases（①－⑥）with the correct definitions (meaning 'in context') from the box below (a－f). Also choose the appropriate Japanese translation（ア－カ）for each term.

下の語（句）は、すべて **STORY** に出てくるものです。それぞれの英語の説明として、ふさわしいものをa～fの中から選びなさい。さらにその日本語の意味として、最もふさわしいものをア～カの中から選びなさい。

① necessitate　　（　）（　）　　② sense of identity　（　）（　）
③ virulent　　　 （　）（　）　　④ critical period　　（　）（　）

⑤ anachronism ( ) ( )　　　⑥ experiential　　( ) ( )

> a) based on or relating to experience
> b) awareness of self
> c) the specific period in which the important events in question occur
> d) very dangerous in effects
> e) someone or something that belongs to a period other than that in which it exists
> f) make necessary

ア　臨界期（ある反応について重要な一定時期）　　イ　～を必要とする
ウ　伝染性の強い、命にかかわる　　　　　　　　　エ　時代遅れの人（もの）
オ　同一性意識、自我意識　　　　　　　　　　　　カ　経験上の、経験的な

III COMPREHENSION

The story below will help you to understand Dr. Sacks' patient, Rose. Please read and answer the true or false questions below.

次の英文を読んで、正しいものには T、間違っているものには F をつけましょう。

STORY　　　　　　　　　　　　　　　　　　　　　CD 12

　　Rose was born in New York City in 1905, the youngest child of a large, wealthy, and talented family. Rose grew up happily, surrounded by a loving family, and she had a strong sense of identity. Rose was generally very healthy during her early childhood and school years.

　　On leaving school, she threw herself ardently into an active and vibrant social life. Between 1922 and 1926, Rose experienced more than most people do in all their lives. For example, she flew to various places all over the US and enjoyed a very active 'party life.' In 1926, this suddenly ended when she was struck down by a virulent form of encephalitis lethargica. Three or four years after the initial symptoms, signs of parkinsonism began to manifest themselves. She became rigid, and lost her balance when walking. These symptoms gradually worsened, necessitating full time-nursing care and she was finally admitted to Mount Carmel in 1935.

　　Rose's condition remained unchanged after the age of thirty, and when Dr. Sacks first saw her in 1966, he agreed with the original notes from her admission. She displayed profuse drooling, global akinesia, intense axial rigidity, and was in near-continuous oculogyric crisis. Rose had a minimal capacity to speak or move and this ability disappeared altogether during her more severe crises. Her most severe crises were associated with pain, which coalesced with feelings of dread and threat.

Dr. Sacks could not make up his mind about whether or not to use L-dopa on Rose when the drug became available. She had been almost helpless for about forty years and Dr. Sacks had never seen a patient who inhabited such an 'inaccessible world of her own.' Rose's unique and complex situation made Dr. Sacks wonder and even fear what might happen if she received L-dopa.

Nevertheless, Dr. Sacks started Rose on L-dopa, despite his misgivings, in the middle of June 1969. Rose displayed the first therapeutic responses a week later, even though the dosage was only 1.5 grams a day, In fact, by this stage, Rose had experienced two full days without any apparent oculogyric crises. By the first of July, she began to speak in a normal conversational volume and was able to walk without assistance. Rose now began receiving 4 grams of L-dopa and she continued to improve. She was actively mobile and was delighted with the results of the L-dopa treatment.

Things did not continue forever in this positive direction. By the beginning of July, the L-dopa treatment's effectiveness began to decline. Over the next month, Rose exhibited mood swings, displayed tics, suffered grave changes in her ability to walk and talk, and endured several oculogyric crises. By August, only a few positive effects of the L-dopa were apparent.

During the critical period in July 1969, Dr. Sacks observed a strange state of nostalgia in Rose. As Rose was able to talk to Dr. Sacks, he was able to understand that even in her 'nostalgic' state, she was completely aware that it was 1969 and that she was sixty-four years old, but that she felt like she was still in 1926 and only twenty-one years old. However, she added that she was not able to really imagine what it was like being older than twenty-one, because she had never really experienced it. The L-dopa must have de-blocked Rose for a few days and exposed this strange anachronism relating to the almost fifty year gap between her biological and experiential age.

Rose was in a sense a 'Sleeping Beauty' whose 'awakening' was hard for her to handle. To deal with this, she apparently re-blocked herself and consequently prevented the possibility of any similar reaction to L-dopa in the future.

Notes

5 **ardently**「熱心に」   6 **vibrant**「活気に満ちた」   9 **be struck down**「（病気）に襲われる」   10 **initial symptom(s)**「初期症状」   11 **manifest oneself**「（兆候が）現われる」   17 **admission**「入院」   17 **profuse drooling**「おびただしくよだれが出ること」   17 **global akinesia**「全体的無動」   17-**intense axial rigidity**「体幹部の重い固縮」   18 **oculogyric crisis**「注視発症、注視痙攣、注視クリーゼ」嗜眠性脳炎、フェニチアジンによる眼球の上方回転発作。   18-**minimal capacity**「最小限の能力」   21 **coalesce with**「〜と連合する、一緒になる」   21 **dread and threat**「恐怖と脅かし」   25 **inhabit**「〜に住む」   25 **'inaccessible world of one's own'**「自分だけの誰も入り込めない世界」   29 **misgiving**「不安、懸念」   32 **apparent**「明らかな」   33 **conversational volume**「会話のできる声量」   40 **grave**「深刻な」   45 **'nostalgic' state**「回想している間、状態」   50 **de-block**「妨害から開放する」   53 **'Sleeping Beauty'**「眠れる森の美女」   54 **re-block**「再び妨害する」

True or False Questions

1. (　) Dr. Sacks hesitated to give L-dopa to Rose, because it was difficult for him to predict what would happen if she took the drug.
2. (　) Rose was put in the hospital soon after she was diagnosed with encephalitis lethargica.
3. (　) The last year in which Rose 'really lived' was 1926, when she was twenty one.
4. (　) Rose was very sure that she was twenty-one after she awoke in July 1969.
5. (　) Rose was happy with L-dopa, around the first of July, soon after her treatment began.

Ⅳ USEFUL EXPRESSIONS

The following sentences were used in Dr. Sacks' original book. Use the hints below to help you to accurately translate the sentences into Japanese.

次の英文は、すべてサックス博士の小説 ***Awakenings*** に出てくるものです。それぞれの語（句）の注を参考に、日本語に訳してみましょう。

1. …., she <u>steered clear of</u> <u>significant neurotic problems</u> or '<u>identity crises</u>' <u>in her growing-up period</u>.

steer clear of ～「～をうまく切り抜ける」　**significant neurotic problem(s)**「重大な精神的問題」　**'identity crisis'**（**pl. crises**）「アイデンティティの危機」　**in one's growing-up period**「～が成長期に」

2. And this was as well, for at the age of twenty-one she <u>was suddenly struck down by</u> a <u>virulent form</u> of encephalitis lethargica—one of its last victims <u>before the epidemic vanished</u>.

   be struck down by ～「～（病気などに）に襲われる」　**virulent form**「伝染力の高い型（病原型）」　**before the epidemic vanish(ed)**「大流行が終結する前」

3. Keep her quiet and feed her—<u>she'll be fine in</u> a week.

   S will be fine in ～「Sは～で良くなるでしょう」

4. Her energy seems limitless and untiring, although I <u>get the impression of</u> exhaustion somewhere beneath the <u>pressured surface</u>.

   get the impression of ～「～の印象を受ける」　**pressured surface**「押さえられた表面」

5. She continues to look much younger than her years; indeed, <u>in a fundamental sense</u>, she is much younger than her age.

   in a fundamental sense「本質的に」

46

Ⅴ LISTENING FOCUS　　　　　　　　　　　　　　　　　　　CD 13

Please listen to Chapter 6-Dialog 6 and fill in the blanks with appropriate words, expressions, or phrases.

次の会話を聞いて、空欄の英語を聞き取ってみましょう。

Dialog 6

Dr. Sacks: What're you thinking about, Rose?
Rose: Nothing, nothing.
Dr. Sacks: But how (　　　)(　　　)(　　　)(　　　) thinking of nothing?
Rose: It's dead easy, once you know how.
Dr. Sacks: So how exactly do (　　　)(　　　)(　　　)(　　　)?
Rose: I think of positive nothings and negative (　　　).
Dr. Sacks: And what are those like?
Rose: That's impossible to say because when I think of a thought, it's suddenly gone. Sometimes I think of a picture in my mind then (　　　)(　　　)(　　　) as fast as I can make it.

Ⅵ MORE ABOUT AMERICAN HEALTH ISSUES

アメリカの病院－その歴史2　History of American Hospitals (part 2)

　1800年頃までに発展したボランタリー病院は、裕福で権力のあるスポンサーの寄付から成り立っており、患者の治療費もそのほとんどを無料で提供するところが多かった。このため、高額の寄付提供者の発言力は医師より大きく、病院経営への関与もまた大きかった。1800年代中期になると、カソリック系の移民が増え、宗教系の病院も設立され始めた。また、寄付に頼らない営利病院も出現し始めた。1900年代には、産業の発展とともに、営利病院が急成長するところとなり、小規模でも手術センターとしての役割を持ち、運営資金を裕福な患者の治療費でまかなうところも多かった。

　現在のコミュニティー病院の8割は歴史的に慈善を目的として発展した自治体病院とボランタリー病院で占められている。自治体病院やボランタリー病院と営利病院は、その目的と成り立ちの違いから、現在でもその経営方針や組織構造にも違いが見られる。この話の舞台であるマウント・カーメル病院は、自治体病院を母体としたコミュニティー病院である。

Ⅶ YOUR OPINIONS

次の英語の質問に対し、英語または日本語で答えてみましょう。さらに、グループで話し合ってみるのもよいでしょう。

Q1. What do you think of the strange sense of nostalgia Rose exhibited after awakening?

Q2. Was Rose's background an important factor in the outcome of her treatment?

Ⅷ MEDICAL ENGLISH ENHANCER（英語で調べてみよう）

Complete a short (5-6 sentences) summary of the following medical term(s). Use English references as your source material.

"coping mechanism"（対処メカニズム）について英語の文献で調べ、それを5行程度の英文でまとめてみましょう。それを参考にローズにL-dopaが効かなくなった要因について考えてみましょう。

Chapter 7
Hester Y. (1)

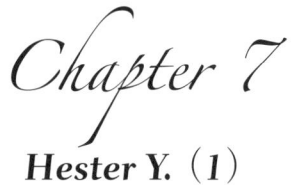

　19歳で結婚したヘスターは、二人の子供にも恵まれて10年ほどは平穏に暮らしていました。しかし、次第に体に変調をきたし、ついに家族と離れ、36歳のときにマウント・カーメルに入院しました。そこでサックス医師と出会い、L-dopaの治療を受けることになるのです。

I PRE-READING
Absence Epilepsy（欠神癲癇）

The following information on 'absence epilepsy' will help you to understand how the original diagnosis for this patient, Hester, was formed.

Fact 1: People with absence epilepsy have repeated seizures that cause momentary lapses of consciousness and so these are described as "absence seizures".

Fact 2: Absence epilepsy is often characterized by age of onset, e. g., childhood absence epilepsy for epilepsy beginning in childhood between the ages of three and twelve.

Fact 3: Absence epilepsy tends to run in families, suggesting it may have genetic components.

II VOCABULARY & IDIOMATIC EXPRESSIONS

The following terms are used in the story below. Match each of the following words or phrases (①-⑥) with the correct definitions (meaning 'in context') from the box below (a-f). Also choose the appropriate Japanese translation (ア-カ) for each term.

下の語（句）は、すべて **STORY** に出てくるものです。それぞれの英語の説明として、ふさわしいものをa～fの中から選びなさい。さらにその日本語の意味として、最もふさわしいものをア～カの中から選びなさい。

① abrupt　　　　　（　）（　）　② interruption　　　　（　）（　）
③ foundation　　　（　）（　）　④ halt　　　　　　　　（　）（　）
⑤ decomposition　（　）（　）　⑥ be institutionalized　（　）（　）

a) bring or come to a sudden stop
b) someone that serves as the base or source of strength in a group
c) stop the continuous progress of an activity or process
d) breaking down; becoming ineffective
e) be placed or kept in a residential institution for medical care
f) sudden and unexpected

ア　分解　　　　　　　　イ　〈精神病患者・アルコール中毒患者などを〉施設に収容する
ウ　急の、突然の　　　　　エ　（行動・活動が）止まる、停止する
オ　土台、よりどころ　　　カ　遮られた状態、中断

III COMPREHENSION

The story below will help you to understand Dr. Sacks' patient, Hester. Please read and answer the true or false questions below.

次の英文を読んで、正しいものにはT、間違っているものにはFをつけましょう。

STORY — CD 14

　　Born in Brooklyn, Hester was an intelligent, independent woman who had married at nineteen and quickly had two children. For ten years after her marriage, she enjoyed her family life. With her special personality and nature, she functioned as the foundation on which the family was built. Her disease changed all of that.

　　At first, her symptoms were bizarre and paroxysmal. She would suddenly halt whatever she was doing such as walking and talking. These interruptions, which were considered to be caused by a kind of absence epilepsy, gradually became longer and occasionally lasted for several hours. As these symptoms evolved, her doctors changed their diagnosis of her condition to 'hysteria.'

　　After two years of paroxysmal standstills, parkinsonian signs appeared, along with indications of catatonia or trance, and all speech and thought were impeded. She was almost completely immobile and speechless by her thirty-fifth year and finally had to be institutionalized at Mount Carmel when she was thirty-six years old. After her entry into Mt. Carmel, Hester's family literally broke apart—Hester's husband divorced her after just two visits to Mt. Carmel, her daughter developed acute psychosis, and her son left for the west somewhere.

At Mount Carmel, despite her extreme immobility, her humor shone through and she was popular among the staff and patients. In May 1969, since Dr. Sacks was concerned about Hester dying from starvation, he decided to use L-dopa as a life-saving measure and the drug was first administered, in orange-juice, on May 7.

Although the daily L-dopa dosage was increased to 4 grams during the first ten days, Hester showed no change at all. On May 16, Dr. Sacks began to administer L-dopa in apple sauce to avoid any possible decomposition of the drug in the acidic orange-juice. The next day, Hester suddenly started walking around the hospital, talking to everyone. She didn't slowly 'warm up' as the other patients did, but rather her awakening was so abrupt that the nurses described it as an 'explosion.'

Notes

6 **bizarre**「〈外観・様式・性質などが〉怪奇な、奇異な」　6 **paroxysmal**「(感情・行動などが突然に) 激発する、発作的な」　8-**absence epilepsy**「〔病理〕欠神癲癇（てんかん）」　11 '**hysteria**'「ヒステリー症」神経症の一種で激しい感情爆発、知覚・運動機能の障害などの異常を特徴とする　12 **paroxysmal standstill**「発作性の停止症状」　13 **indication**「徴候」　13 **catatonia**「〔精神医学〕緊張病、緊張型分裂病、カタトニー」精神分裂症（**schizophrenia**）の一型に見られる症候群　13 **trance**「夢うつつ、意識もうろう」　18-**acute psychosis**「急性の精神病」高度の精神機能障害で、現実への適応能力が著しく欠如した状態　20-**shine through**「はっきり分かる、ありありと見える」　22 **starvation**「飢餓（状態）」　28 **acidic**「酸性の」　31 '**explosion**'「爆発」

True or False Questions

1. (　) Hester had been the foundation of her family because of her strong character.
2. (　) Dr. Sacks decided to give Hester L-dopa because he feared that she would die from starvation.
3. (　) Before Hester came to Mount Carmel, her doctors had only diagnosed her with a kind of absence epilepsy.
4. (　) Since Hester had strong family ties, her family members continuously supported her stay at Mount Carmel.
5. (　) Like all the other L-dopa recipients, Hester responded immediately to the treatment.

IV USEFUL EXPRESSIONS

The following sentences were used in Dr. Sacks' original book. Use the hints below to help you to accurately translate the sentences into Japanese.

次の英文は、すべてサックス博士の小説 ***Awakenings*** に出てくるものです。それぞれの語（句）の注を参考に、日本語に訳してみましょう。

1. Hester was born in Brooklyn, the elder child of an immigrant couple. She had no illnesses of note in her growing-up years, certainly nothing which suggested encephalitis lethargica.

   (the) elder child of an immigrant couple「移民の夫婦の年長の子」　**have no illnesses of note in one's growing-up years**「成長期に注意する病気かからない」　**which suggests encephalitis lethargica**「嗜眠性脳炎と思われる〜」

2. She took everything in her stride. And she could laugh at everything, especially herself.

   take 〜 in one's stride「〜を難なく切り抜ける」　**laugh at everything**「何でも笑い飛ばす」

3. It is clear that Hester was the fulcrum of her family, giving it balance and stability with her own strength of character, and that when she became ill, its foundations were rocked.

   (the) fulcrum of one's family「家族の支え」　**give 〜 balance and stability**「〜にバランスと安定を与える」　**its foundations are rocked**「その礎(いしずえ)が揺れ動かされる」

4. Her husband visited her twice in hospital, and found it unbearable; he never came again, and finally divorced her.

find it unbearable「それが耐え難いことがわかる」　**finally divorce her**「ついに彼女と離婚する」

5. Fearing that some or all of the drug <u>was being decomposed by the acid[ic] orange-juice</u> in which it was being given, <u>I requested</u>, on 16 May, <u>that it be given in apple sauce instead</u>.

---

be decomposed by the acid[ic] orange-juice「酸性のオレンジジュースで分解される」　**S request that it (should) be given in apple sauce instead**「S が（それを）代わりにアップルソースと一緒に与えるように要求する」

V LISTENING FOCUS　　　　　　　　　　　　　　　CD 15

Please listen to Chapter 7-Dialog 7 and fill in the blanks with appropriate words, expressions, or phrases.

次の会話を聞いて、空欄の英語を聞き取ってみましょう。

Dialog 7

Nurse:　You look wonderful today, Hester.
Hester:　Yes. I'm (　　　)(　　　)(　　　)(　　　).
Nurse:　Enjoy yourself. Is everything okay?
Hester:　Well, I had a bit of a spell this morning. My brother was visiting and well, it happened again. I (　　　)(　　　)(　　　).
Nurse:　(　　　)(　　　)(　　　)(　　　)?
Hester:　Well, he lit a match to light his pipe and it turns out I saw him light the pipe before he did it. It's that strange freeze frame vision I get.
Nurse:　(　　　)(　　　)(　　　)(　　　)(　　　).
Hester:　No. There are too many things to do and my daughter is coming tomorrow. I want to tell her all about the concert.

VI MORE ABOUT AMERICAN HEALTH ISSUES

言語聴覚士（言語療法士）（Speech-Language Therapist）と視能訓練士（Optometrist）

　言語聴覚士は、音声機能、言語機能、摂食・嚥下機能、又は聴覚に障害のある人に対し、医師又は歯科医師の指示のもとに、検査、評価を行い、その機能の維持向上を図るために訓練や指導、そして援助を行う。視能訓練士は、視機能の検査（視力、視野、屈折、色覚、眼圧など）や、斜視や弱視の視力回復治療などを行う。また、視能訓練士は眼科医の指導のもとに基礎データを出し、訓練プログラムをたて、視機能回復のための訓練を行なう。日本では両者とも、大学や専門教育機関を卒業して国家試験を受験する資格を得、国家試験に合格することが必要である。合格し、その資格を得ると、教育機関、保健福祉機関、医療機関で幅広く活動できる。

　一方、アメリカでは、言語聴覚士は、単独で患者の診断と治療に当たることができるが、大学院の修士課程を卒業しなければ国家試験を受けることができない。視能訓練士も大学を卒業することが必要とされている。

VII YOUR OPINIONS

次の英語の質問に対し、英語または日本語で答えてみましょう。後で、グループで話し合ってみるのも良いでしょう。

Q. We saw that Hester's family broke apart after she was admitted to Mt. Carmel. Clearly the family was traumatized by the loss of a central familial figure. Do you think this is a common problem with patients? If so, should the care of any patient also involve counseling for the patient's immediate family?

_____

_____

_____

_____

_____

_____

Chapter 8
Hester Y. (2)

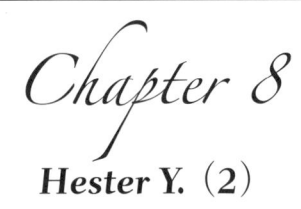

　ヘスターはL-dopaの複雑な副作用にも耐え、L-dopaを服用しながらマウント・カーメルで友人に恵まれた生活を送り続けました。彼女は発病して入院したことによって失ってしまった息子や娘とも、治療後には再会することができました。さて、なぜそれが可能となったのでしょうか。

I PRE-READING
Tic-like Movements（チック）

The following information on 'tic-like movements' will help you to understand how the original diagnosis for this patient, Hester, was formed.

Fact 1: A tic is a sudden, repetitive, stereotyped, non-rhythmic, involuntary movement (motor tic) or sound (phonic tic) that involves discrete groups of muscles.

Fact 2: Tics are generally classified as motor vs. phonic and simple vs. complex.

Fact 3: Tics can be invisible to the observer (e.g.; abdominal tensing or toe crunching).

Fact 4: Motor aspects of other movement disorders (e.g.; chorea, dystonia, myoclonus) must be distinguished from tics. Other conditions (e.g.; autism, stereotypic movement disorder) also include movements which may be confused with tics.

Fact 5: Tics must also be distinguished from the compulsions of obsessive compulsive disorder and from seizure activity.

II VOCABULARY & IDIOMATIC EXPRESSIONS

The following terms are used in the story below. Match each of the following words or phrases (①−⑥) with the correct definitions (meaning 'in context') from the box below (a−f). Also choose the appropriate Japanese translation (ア−カ) for each term.

　下の語（句）は、すべて **STORY** に出てくるものです。それぞれの英語の説明として、ふさわしいものをa～fの中から選びなさい。さらにその日本語の意味として、最もふさわしいものをア～カの中から選びなさい。

① remarkable　　　　　　(　)(　)　② revert　　　　(　)(　)
③ become accustomed to (　)(　)　④ extravagant　(　)(　)
⑤ unpredictable　　　　　(　)(　)　⑥ astound　　　(　)(　)

> a) to become used to something
> b) excessive, not showing restraint, extreme
> c) return to a previous state, practice, topic, etc.
> d) to make someone very surprised or shocked
> e) something that cannot be estimated/specified in the future
> f) worthy of attention; striking

ア　〜に慣れる、〜が習慣化する　　イ　（元の状態などに）戻る
ウ　途方も無い、とっぴな　　　　　エ　注目すべき、注目に値する
オ　予測できない、変わりやすい　　カ　びっくり仰天させる

III COMPREHENSION

The story below will help you to understand Dr. Sacks' patient, Hester. Please read and answer the true or false questions below.

次の英文を読んで、正しいものにはT、間違っているものにはFをつけましょう。

STORY　　　　　　　　　　　　　　　　　　　　　　　　CD 16

　　Although Hester's 'explosive' response to L-dopa seemed to be positive, after a few days she started to have compulsive tic-like movements and excitable and hysterical behaviors, compelling Dr. Sacks to gradually lower her dose to 1 gram/day. On May 24, Hester asked Dr. Sacks to stop the L-dopa, claiming that it was too much for her to handle. Dr. Sacks complied, and by the next day, Hester had reverted to being motionless and speechless again. Dr. Sacks was astounded that Hester's whole triumphant emergence, 'complications,' and withdrawal, had all taken place within a single week.

　　Hester continued to take L-dopa after 1969. Forty months after May 25, Dr. Sacks characterized Hester, among all his patients, as the one who displayed the most extravagant and unstable physiological activities and reactions to L-dopa. For example, Hester became so sensitive to L-dopa (her dose was decreased to 750 mg/day) that whenever the drug administration was stopped, she immediately fell into a coma. Moreover,

Hester also experienced periods—usually unpredictable in duration, onset, and cessation—during which her movements, speech, and thoughts seemed almost normal. Nevertheless, Dr. Sacks believed that Hester was also the 'coolest' in handling, diverting, and managing these excessive side-effects. In fact, she became accustomed to all of these strange reactions and handled them well, using her innate strength and positive spirit.

Hester was always active in and out of the hospital, and managed as full a life as could be expected at Mount Carmel. The final source of Hester's strength—as with so many patients—seems to have come from personal relations; in her case reunions with her son and daughter whom she had not seen in fifteen years or more.

Thus, Hester would seem to have been a successful L-dopa patient. Despite her continuously excessive reactions to L-dopa, she nevertheless has remained awake with the treatment, has returned to reality, and has achieved a remarkable improvement. Nobody could have imagined that such a recovery was possible.

Notes

2-**compulsive tic-like movement**「チックに似た衝動的な動き」　3 **excitable and hysterical behavior**「興奮し理性のなくなった行動」　3 **compel**「〈人に〉無理やり~させる」　6 **comply**「(希望や要求などに) 従う」　8 **triumphant**「〈人・事が〉勝利を収めた、成功した」　8 '**complications**'「〔病理〕(はじめの病気を悪化させる) 合併症、併発症」　8 **withdrawal**「(薬物の) 禁断状態」　12 **physiological activity**「生理 (的) 活動」　15 **coma**「昏睡」　16 **duration**「継続期間」　17 **onset**「始まり」　17 **cessation**「休止、停止、中断」　19 **divert**「気晴らしをする」　21 **innate strength**「生来の強さ」ここで **strength** は精神力の強さを意味する。　26 **reunion**「再会、和解」

True or False Questions

1. (　) Hester's unique characteristics allowed her to adapt to her violent over-reactions to the L-dopa treatment .
2. (　) Dr. Sacks was forced to reduce Hester's dose of L-dopa because she started to have compulsive tic-like movements.
3. (　) Hester was unhappy when she met her daughter and son after an interval of more than fifteen years.
4. (　) No one, including Dr. Sacks, expected Hester's remarkable recovery.
5. (　) Like other patients, Hester showed unexpected and unstable reactions to L-dopa.

IV USEFUL EXPRESSIONS

The following sentences were used in Dr. Sacks' original book. Use the hints below to help you to accurately translate the sentences into Japanese.

次の英文は、すべてサックス博士の小説 *Awakenings* に出てくるものです。それぞれの語（句）の注を参考に、日本語に訳してみましょう。

1. Her writings, at this time, were almost entirely expressions of blame, rage and terror, mingled with feelings of grief and loss.

   expression(s) of blame, rage and terror「責め、怒りそして恐怖の表現」
   (be) mingled with feelings of ～「～の感情が混じる」

2. It has been indicated that within three days of her 'awakening' on L-dopa, Hester showed the onset of clear-cut tics.

   (the) onset of clear-cut ～「明白な～の開始」

3. Her daughter, who had spend two decades in and out of mental hospitals since Hester became ill, is now a frequent and much-loved visitor at Mount Carmel.

   two decades「20年間」　**in and out of** ～「～を出たり入ったりする」
   much-loved visitor「誰からも好かれる訪問者」

4. Seeing Hester with her son and daughter, one realizes the strength of her character and love; one sees what a remarkable person she is, and how solid and real she must have been as a mother.

(the) strength of her character and love 「彼女の性格と愛情の強さ」 **how solid and real she must have been as a mother** 「彼女がいかに母親としてしっかりしていて現実的であったか」

Ⅴ LISTENING FOCUS 　　　　　　　　　　　　　　　　　CD 17

Please listen to Chapter 8-Dialog 8 (the text is reproduced below) and fill in the blanks with appropriate words, expressions, or phrases.

次の会話を聞いて、空欄の英語を聞き取ってみましょう。

Dialog 8

Dr. Sacks is playing ball with Hester and his students. One of Hester's symptoms is her accelerated behavior. Her movements are too powerful and energetic. Hester apparently does not know how strong and quick her reaction time is when playing ball.

Dr. Sacks:　Would you like to play a game with my students, Hester?
Hester:　　Of course! (　　　)(　　　)(　　　)(　　　)!
Student A:　Wow!　It's impossible to catch her throws. I cannot believe how strong and fast she is!
Dr. Sacks:　You see (　　　) (　　　) (　　　) (　　　). Don't underestimate her—you'd better be ready.
Student B:　Hester, you have to slow down! (　　　)(　　　)(　　　)(　　　), and then throw it back.
Hester:　　O.K., no problem!
[Short pause]
Student B:　Hey!　I (　　　) you (　　　) (　　　) (　　　)(　　　)!
Hester:　　But I *did* count to ten!

Ⅵ MORE ABOUT AMERICAN HEALTH ISSUES

理学療法士（Physical Therapist／Physiotherapist）と作業療法士（Occupational Therapist）

　日本の理学療法士は、医師の指示のもとで高齢者や交通事故など後天的な、または新生児の運動能力の発達の遅れなど先天的な身体機能障害のある人に対して機能回復を促したり、自立生活への手助けをする。歩行、車椅子の訓練などの運動療法や、日常生活動作訓練、マッサージ療法などを行い、回復に導く。作業療法士は、身体または精神に障害のある人やまたはそれが予測される人に対し、リハビリテーションとして、その応用的動作能力又は社会的適応能力を、手芸、工作その他の作業によって、回復を図るものである。両者とも大学・専門学校教育によって養成され、その卒業時に国家試験の受験資格を得、試験に合格すると、それぞれ理学療法士、作業療法士として各種病院や施設などで治療に従事することができる。

　一方、アメリカの理学療法士は、国家試験を受ける資格として、少なくとも大学院の修士課程を卒業していることが必要で、博士課程までのコースを用意する教育養成機関も多く、より高度な知識と技術を要求され、国家試験に合格すると、単独で患者の診断と治療に当たる。作業療法士も大学を卒業する必要があるが、最近は修士や博士課程を卒業していることが望まれてきている。

Ⅶ YOUR OPINIONS

次の英語の質問に対し、英語または日本語で答えてみましょう。さらに、グループで話し合ってみるのもよいでしょう。

Q. Hester used her innate strengths to adapt to the wildly oscillating effects of the treatment process. Do all people possess this ability?

　　_____

　　How can patients be helped to mine or access their inner strength?

　　_____

　　_____

　　_____

　　_____

Ⅷ MEDICAL ENGLISH ENHANCER（英語で調べてみよう）

Complete a short (5-6 sentences) summary of the following medical term(s). Use English references as your source material.

"placebo effects"（プラシーボ効果）について英語の文献で調べ、それを5行程度の英文でまとめてみましょう。それを参考にヘスターが回復した要因について考えてみましょう。

Chapter 9
Rolando P.

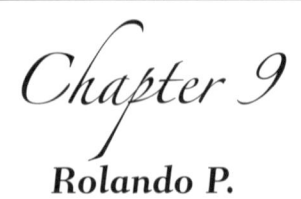

　ロランドはわずか2歳半で嗜眠性脳炎を患い、15年間を自宅で母親とともに過ごし、18歳でマウント・カーメルに入院しました。その後は穏やかな患者として入院生活を送っていましたが、サックス医師と出会い、L-dopa を服用することになります。彼には「目覚め」が訪れるのでしょうか。

I PRE-READING

Euthanasia（安楽死）

Please choose the most appropriate answers ((a) – (d)) for the following statements.

Euthanasia is also sometimes called (①　　　　　). This is a problem that doctors all over the world struggle with. Various classifications—voluntary or (②　　　　), passive or (③　　　　)—have been used to try to categorize this controversial practice, and some medical professionals distinguish between withholding treatment to allow a patient to die as opposed to killing a patient by a deliberate act. The 'Do Not Resuscitate' (DNR) orders are a very specific and less controversial type of guideline used in these situations. (④　　　　), which instruct doctors not to take any extraordinary measures to revive patients whose hearts have stopped, are becoming quite common in many parts of the world.

(a)　involuntary　　(b)　'assisted suicide'
(c)　DNRs　　　　 (d)　active

II VOCABULARY & IDIOMATIC EXPRESSIONS

The following terms are used in the story below. Match each of the following words or phrases (①–⑥) with the correct definitions (meaning 'in context') from the box below (a–f). Also choose the appropriate Japanese translation (ア–カ) for each term.

　下の語（句）は、すべて **STORY** に出てくるものです。それぞれの英語の説明として、ふさわしいものをa～fの中から選びなさい。さらにその日本語の意味として、最もふさわしいものをア～カの中から選びなさい。

① regimen　　　（ ）（ ）　　② overshadow　　　　　　（ ）（ ）
③ pronounced　（ ）（ ）　　④ intensely　　　　　　　（ ）（ ）
⑤ unstable　　（ ）（ ）　　⑥ therapeutic compromise（ ）（ ）

> a) therapy in which the positive effects of a treatment are balanced against its negative effects
> b) a prescribed course of medical treatment to promote or restore health
> c) with extreme force, degree, or strength
> d) very obvious or noticeable
> e) when one thing, out of a group, becomes more important or significant (especially by becoming more noticeable) than the others
> f) likely to change suddenly and perhaps become worse

ア　変わりやすい、不安定な　　イ　治療的妥協点　　ウ　覆い隠す、圧倒する
エ　処方（投薬）計画　　　　　オ　強烈に、きわめて激しく
カ　はっきりした、目立つ

III COMPREHENSION

The story below will help you to understand Dr. Sacks' patient, Rolando. Please read and answer the true or false questions below.

次の英文を読んで、正しいものにはT、間違っているものにはFをつけましょう。

STORY　　　　　　　　　　　　　　　　　　　　　　　　CD 18

　　The youngest son of a newly immigrated Italian family, Rolando was born in New York in 1917. He was active, affectionate, and talkative, until he was thirty months old, when he was struck by encephalitis lethargica, the worst symptoms of which lasted eighteen weeks. After he awoke, he had an expressionless face, had great difficulty in moving or talking, and his schooling suffered greatly. In 1935, he began his stay at Mount Carmel where, except for brief periods of movement and speech, he just sat in his chair all day like a statue.

　　Dr. Sacks examined Rolando and talked to him several times between 1966 and 1969. Although Rolando looked much younger than his actual age, he was one of the most profoundly disabled post-encephalitic (PE) patients Dr. Sacks had ever seen. Dr. Sacks started him on L-dopa on May 14, 1969. Rolando started to respond to the drug one week later, when the L-dopa dosage was 3 grams/day. He lost a lot of the rigidity he had previously suffered; he began to speak, to make fists, and he was even able to stride around the ward, albeit with some assistance. Because of some side effects, mostly involving excessive arousal, Dr. Sacks reduced the L-dopa dose, a few days later, from 3 grams/day to 2 grams/day.

In June, Rolando exhibited major new symptoms involving increased stimulation, agitation, anxiety, and irritability. Dr. Sacks tried to control Rolando's excitomotor syndrome first by reducing the L-dopa to 1.5 grams/day, and then by adding 1.5 mg/day of haloperidol. But, because the symptoms continued, Dr. Sacks finally settled on a regimen of 1 gram L-dopa/day together with the haloperidol.

By mid-July, Dr. Sacks faced the same problem with Rolando's case that he had seen in all the other very severe PE parkinsonism patients: how exactly to treat patients with exceedingly unstable nervous systems and behaviors characterized by oscillatory, bi-polar, and all-or-none features. Dr. Sacks used the same overall strategy for Rolando—one of therapeutic compromise—that he had used for his other patients. Hence, Rolando continued to take 1 gram of L-dopa daily; if he missed a dose he became deeply disabled, and if he missed a day he went into a stupor or coma. From 1970, Rolando's reactions to L-dopa became less pronounced, in that his parkinsonian periods came to overshadow his excited-expansive states.

Rolando enjoyed his best moods and functioning when his family took him home for occasional weekends or holidays but he was always intensely depressed when he returned from the country.

Notes

2 **affectionate**「愛情深い、優しい」 2 **talkative**「おしゃべりな」 5 **expressionless**「〈声・顔などが〉表情のない、表情に乏しい」 14 **rigidity**「硬直」 16 **stride around** ～「～を大股で歩き回る」 16 **albeit**「～ではあるが」 17 **arousal**「喚起、覚醒」 20 **agitation**「感情の揺れ、動揺」 21 **excitomotor syndrome**「運動機能促進症候群」 22 **haloperidol**「ハロペリドール（**HLD**）」主要な抗精神病薬；統合失調症、重篤な不安症などの治療に用いる。 23 **settle on** ～「～に決める」 27 **exceedingly**「非常に」 28 **oscillatory**「振動性の」 28 **bi-polar**「両極端の、正反対の」 28-**all-or-none feature**「全てか無の特質」 33 **stupor**「麻痺状態」 35 **excited-expansive state**「興奮した誇大妄想的な状態」 37 **occasional**「時折、たまの」

True or False Questions

1. (　) Rolando was a Parkinson's disease patient.
2. (　) Rolando loved to spend time with his family, and he bitterly resented returning to Mt. Carmel after such trips.
3. (　) Just like the other patients seen so far, Rolando had severe side effects from L-dopa .
4. (　) Rolando's disease caused him to look older than his actual age.
5. (　) Rolando always had a positive attitude about his treatments .

Ⅳ USEFUL EXPRESSIONS

The following sentences were used in Dr. Sacks' original book. Use the hints below to help you to accurately translate the sentences into Japanese.

次の英文は、すべてサックス博士の小説 ***Awakenings*** に出てくるものです。それぞれの語（句）の注を参考に、日本語に訳してみましょう。

1. …., until at thirty months of age his life <u>was</u> suddenly <u>cut across</u> <u>by a virulent attack of</u> encephalitis lethargica, which presented itself as an <u>intense drowsiness</u> lasting eighteen weeks, initially accompanied by high fever and <u>influenzal symptoms</u>.

   _____

   _____

   be cut across「妨げられる」　**by a virulent attack of** ～　「感染力の強い～の発病によって」　**intense drowsiness**「強い嗜眠状態」　**influenzal symptom(s)**「インフルエンザの症状」

2. …., but <u>conveyed to</u> at least one teacher <u>the impression of</u> an intact but <u>imprisoned intelligence</u>; "Rolando is not stupid," said a <u>report</u> in 1925.

   _____

   _____

   convey to「〈～を〉（…に）伝える」　**(the) impression of**「～という印象」　**imprisoned intelligence**「内側に閉じ込められている知性」　**report**「成績評価」

3. <u>Very occasionally</u> he shows a 'normal' or <u>middle state</u>, but these are only seen once or twice a month and then only last <u>a few seconds or minutes</u>.

   _____

very occasionally「非常にまれに」   **middle state**「中間の状態」   **a few seconds or minutes**「2、3秒か2、3分」

4. <u>On several occasions</u>, we have tried the effects of amantadine—which, in some patients, reduces <u>pathological responses to L-dopa</u> and <u>retrieves (if temporarily) its therapeutic effects</u>.

on several occasions「何度か」   **pathological responses to L-dopa**「L-dopaへの病的反応」   **retrieve(s) (if temporarily) its therapeutic effect(s)**「(一時的にせよ) その治療的効果を回復する」

V LISTENING FOCUS — CD 19

Please listen to Chapter 9-Dialog 9 (the text is reproduced below) and fill in the blanks with appropriate words, expressions, or phrases.

次の会話を聞いて、空欄の英語を聞き取ってみましょう。

Dialog 9

Because Rolando always enjoyed his outings to his relative's home in the country, he always exhibited anger and frustration with his life in the institution when he returned to Mount Carmel.

Dr. Sacks: Good afternoon, Rolando. It's a beautiful day! (　　　)(　　　)(　　　)(　　　)(　　　)?

Rolando: It was a goddamn relief to get out of this place. I've been shut up in places since the day I was born.

Dr. Sacks: Rolando, (　　　)(　　　)(　　　)(　　　) to (　　　)(　　　). I thought you were content here.

Rolando: This is a hell of a life for someone to have.

Dr. Sacks: We are trying our best with the L-dopa. (　　　)(　　　)(　　　).

Rolando: I'm sick of L-dopa. What about a real pill from the cupboard that you lock up?

Nurse: Rolando, you worry too much. What are you talking about?

Rolando: I'm talking about the 'euthanazy' pill or whatever it's called … I've needed that pill since (　　　)(　　　) I (　　　)(　　　).

VI MORE ABOUT AMERICAN HEALTH ISSUES

アメリカにおける看護師　Nurses in America

　日本では、婦長、看護師、准看護師と、その役職や名称は分かれているが、基本的にはその仕事の内容に大きな違いがあるとはいえないであろう。しかし、アメリカでは、受けた教育、持っている資格によって、看護師は大きく、NP（Nurse Practitioner）、RN（Registered Nurse）、LPN（Licensed Practical Nurse）の三つに分けられる。いずれも各州政府から免許が交付されるが、仕事内容、権限、そして給与にいたるまで明確に異なっている。NP（上級看護師）は、RN（正看護師）として認められた者で、さらに看護系大学院、あるいは認定プログラムを履修後、資格試験に合格すると、各州政府から免許が交付される。州によっては、医師の監督なしで簡単な治療や投薬の処方権を持ち、また、開業することもできる。RN（正看護師）は、短大あるいは四年制大学で二年以上看護必須科目を履修後、資格試験に合格すると各州政府から免許が交付される。LPN（准看護婦）は、短大、あるいは看護専門学校で一年以上の看護必須科目を履修後、資格試験に合格すると各州政府から免許が交付される。医師や正看護師の監督下で患者看護を行う。

VII YOUR OPINIONS

次の英語の質問に対し、英語または日本語で答えてみましょう。さらに、グループで話し合ってみるのもよいでしょう。

Q. How does the issue of euthanasia overlap with Rolando's suicidal tendencies? Remember that Rolando specifically asked for an 'euthanazy pill.'

_____

_____

_____

_____

VIII MEDICAL ENGLISH ENHANCER（英語で調べてみよう）

Complete a short (8-9 sentences) summary of the following medical term(s). Use English references as your source material.

英語の文献を使って、安楽死"euthanasia"についての定義や国によっての制度の違いを調べ、それを10行程度の英文でまとめてみましょう。

Chapter 10
Miriam H.

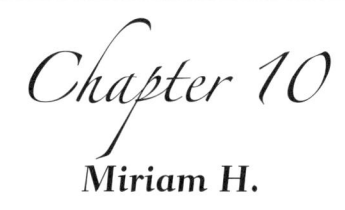

　ミリアムは生後間もない頃から孤児院でつらい日々を過ごしていました。しかし運命は彼女にさらに嗜眠性脳炎という過酷な病を患わせ、彼女はマウント・カーメルへ送られることになりました。やがて L-dopa を服用することにより、特異な才能も示すことになったミリアムは、副作用を克服し、今まで経験したことのない穏やかな日々を送ることができるようになるのです。

I PRE-READING

US Psychiatric Institutions （アメリカの精神病医療の歴史）

In the United States, psychiatric hospitals in the past were often set up as distinct institutions with funding and administrations separate from those of general health care. Since the development of new treatment approaches in the 1950s, there has been an increasing move towards integration of psychiatric treatment within the general health sector.

Please choose the most appropriate answers (from (a) – (f)) for the following statements.

Surgical interventions, known as (①　　　　　), have a long history of use in psychiatry and have gone through several phases. Such treatments were extremely popular in the 1940s. Initially, procedures such as lobotomies were misused but now, in tandem with specialized imaging techniques, such methods have become very useful for some patients in specific situations. Separately, the first (②　　　　　), such as thorazine, became available for the treatment of mental illness in the mid-(③　　　　). These drugs then revolutionized psychiatric care and provided new ways for many of the severely mentally ill to return to normal society. Other new treatments eventually led to reductions in the number of patients in mental hospitals. In the early (④　　　), amid public images of mental hospitals as sites for horror movies, a deinstitutionalisation movement caught hold in many US states. At that time, mental hospitals were viewed as the least desirable solution, both from a humane point of view and from an economic one, to the problem of mental illness.

(a) 1960s　　　　　　(b) 1950s　　　　　(c) psychosurgeries

(d) psychiatric drugs   (e) institutions   (f) psychiatrists

II VOCABULARY & IDIOMATIC EXPRESSIONS

The following terms are used in the story below. Match each of the following words or phrases (①−⑥) with the correct definitions (meaning 'in context') from the box below (a−f). Also choose the appropriate Japanese translation (ア−カ) for each term.

下の語（句）は、すべて **STORY** に出てくるものです。それぞれの英語の説明として、ふさわしいものをa〜fの中から選びなさい。さらにその日本語の意味として、最もふさわしいものをア〜カの中から選びなさい。

① orphanage (　)(　)　② impatient (　)(　)
③ intact   (　)(　)　④ go downhill (　)(　)
⑤ motivation (　)(　)　⑥ fortuitously (　)(　)

> a) not broken or damaged; usually after something bad has happened or after a traumatic experience
> b) to become worse, often used to describe the condition of something
> c) the eagerness or willingness to do something
> d) happening by chance or luck, rather than by intention
> e) a residence for children who cannot be looked after by their parents
> f) very eager for something to happen and not wanting to wait

ア　損なわれていない、変わっていない　　イ　しきりに〜したがる、せっかちな
ウ　思いがけなく、偶然に　　　　　　　　エ　悪化する、衰える
オ　孤児院　　　　　　　　　　　　　　　カ　動機、やる気

III COMPREHENSION

The following story will help you understand Dr. Sacks' patient, Miriam. Please read and answer the true or false questions below.

次の英文を読んで、正しいものにはT、間違っているものにはFをつけましょう。

STORY

> The second child of a deeply religious Jewish family, Miriam was born in 1914 in New York. Orphaned as a baby, she was sent to an orphanage in Queens where she endured 'Dickensian' conditions. Her bad luck continued when, at the age of eleven she suffered fractures to both legs, her pelvis, and back because she was pushed off a bridge.

Moreover, at age twelve, she was the only one in the orphanage of over 200 children to develop encephalitis lethargica. For six months, she slept all day and night, and had to be awoken for food and other necessities. This was followed, further, by a two year period during which she experienced narcolepsies, sleep-paralyses, nightmares, and sleep-talking. Parkinsonism followed, and this left Miriam with left-sided rigidity, a shrunken left hand, postural abnormalities, and changes in her speech and thought patterns. Nevertheless, Miriam's intellect was intact and she was able to finish high school. By eighteen, however, her physical disabilities had become so severe that she was transferred to Mount Carmel Hospital. She would spend all her life in institutions.

Over the next thirty-seven years her condition went downhill, but Miriam could still walk with the aid of two sticks until 1966. Although a variety of hypothalamic disorders resulting in grotesque physical deformities pushed Miriam into a relative state of isolation, she was surprisingly active in ward and synagogue affairs. A striking change to Miriam's condition followed the hot summer of 1967, during which the hospital stopped her anti-Parkinsonian medication because of the fear of hyperpyrexia and heat-stroke. Consequently, Miriam suffered a neurological and emotional regression, and lost all of her former spirit and motivation. As she sat all day motionless in her chair, she was considered a hopeless 'back-ward' patient.

L-dopa was started on June 18, 1969. No changes were observed in the first week. As the dosage was slowly increased to 4 grams/day, Miriam began to pay attention to her appearance, to keep a diary, and to borrow books from the library—unfortunately, she also became more demanding and impatient. With the aid of physiotherapy, she was able to stand and walk a few steps once again. Her transformation had turned her into a healthy, well-dressed, powdered, and made-up 'swan.'

Because Miriam developed increasingly severe respiratory side effects to L-dopa, the treatment was stopped in December 1969, only to be restarted in February 1970. However, the L-dopa now caused excessive ticcing and Miriam herself asked Dr. Sacks to stop the treatment in July 1970.

In September 1970, Miriam changed her mind and said, "Third time lucky! If you give me L-dopa once again, I promise no complications this time." Dr. Sacks agreed and Miriam continued to take 4 grams/day L-dopa for two years. Fortuitously, Miriam was able to lead an active life, going to the movies, playing bingo, and devoting time to her one remaining sister.

Thus, Miriam has done well. Against all odds, Miriam has managed to lead a real life and face her difficulties head on.

Notes

2 **orphan**「〈子供を〉孤児にする」 3 **'Dickensian' conditions**「ディケンズの小説に出て来るような（悲惨な）状況」 5 **pelvis**「骨盤」 10 **narcolepsy**「発作性睡眠」 10 **sleep-paralysis**「睡眠麻痺状態」 10 **nightmare**「悪夢」 10 **sleep-talking**「寝言」 11 **left-sided rigidity**「左半身硬直」 12 **shrunken left hand**「左手の縮小」 19 **hypothalamic disorder**「視床下部障害」 19-**grotesque physical deformity**「グロテスクな身体的な醜さ」 21 **synagogue affair**「礼拝堂の活動」 24 **hyperpyrexia**「超異常高熱」 24 **heat-stroke**「熱射病、暑気あたり」 27 **'back-ward' patient**「ひきこもった患者」 32 **physiotherapy**「物理［理学］療法」 33 **transformation**「変化」 34 **made-up 'swan'**「成長した白鳥（醜いアヒルの子から）」 35 **severe respiratory side effect**「重症の呼吸器の副作用」 40-**third time lucky**「三度目の正直」 44 **one remaining sister**「一人残っている姉」

True or False Questions

1. (　) When Miriam was twelve, she suffered from Parkinson's disease.
2. (　) Miriam was one of the few L-dopa therapy success stories, particularly over the long-term.
3. (　) Miriam was not seriously disabled before the L-dopa treatment was given to her.
4. (　) Miriam was brought up by a wealthy foster family.
5. (　) Miriam was satisfied with and wished to continue her second L-dopa treatment.

IV USEFUL EXPRESSIONS

The following sentences were used in Dr. Sacks' original book. Use the hints below to help you to accurately translate the sentences into Japanese.

次の英文は、すべてサックス博士の小説 ***Awakenings*** に出てくるものです。それぞれの語（句）の注を参考に、日本語に訳してみましょう。

1. "At first," she said, "I hated everybody, I <u>longed for vengeance</u>. I felt that people round me <u>were somehow responsible for</u> my disease. Then I <u>became resigned to it</u>, and <u>realized that</u> it was a punishment from God."

long for vengeance「仕返しを待ち望む」　**be somehow responsible for** 〜「〜にたいして何かしらの責任がある」　**become resigned to it**「それをあきらめるようになる」　**realize that** 〜「〜だと気がつく」

2. Her rapidity of speech, combined with her rapidity of thought and calculation, makes her <u>more than a match for</u> any of my students. When I ask her, for example, to <u>take 17s away from 1,012</u>, she performs these <u>serial subtractions</u> as fast as she can speak.

more than a match for「〜に匹敵する以上に」　**take 17s away from 1,012**「1,012から17を順に引く」　**serial subtractions**「連続引き算」

3. Her <u>obesity</u>, her <u>acromegaly</u>, and her slightly <u>masked face</u> could easily <u>be overlooked now with</u> her new <u>poise and smartness</u>, and especially when one was listening to her <u>admirably witty and fluent conversation</u>. <u>The Ugly Duckling</u> was nearly a swan.

obesity「肥満」　**acromegaly,**「先端（末端）肥大症」　**masked face**「表情に乏しい顔」　**be overlooked now with**「〜で今や大目に見られる、覆い隠される」　**poise and smartness**「落ち着きと明晰さ」　**admirably witty and fluent conversation**「すばらしく機知に富んで流暢な会話」　**the Ugly Duckling**「みにくいアヒルの子」

4. …she <u>is warmly devoted to</u> her one remaining sister. For most of the day however, Miriam <u>is absorbed in reading</u> and writing.

be warmly devoted to「〜をやさしく気遣う」　**be absorbed in**「〜に没頭している、夢中である」

V LISTENING FOCUS　　　　　　　　　　　　　　　　CD 21

Please listen to Chapter 10-Dialog 10 and fill in the blanks with appropriate words, expressions, or phrases.

次の会話を聞いて、空欄の英語を聞き取ってみましょう。

Dialog 10

Miriam had a compulsion to count and compute. This condition, known as arithmomania, was often observed in the beginning of the epidemic and is also seen in Tourette's patients.

Staff:　　What are you doing, Miriam?
Miriam:　I bet you can't guess (　　　)(　　　)(　　　)(　　　) (　　　) today with the numbers 5 and 8?
Staff:　　No, I can't.
Miriam:　16 cars with both 5 and 8, and 20 cars with only 5, and 31 with only 8.
Staff:　　(　　　)(　　　)(　　　)(　　　) all of that?
Miriam:　No problem. Do you want to know the square root of 58? Or how many words are on the page of the book I'm now reading?
Staff:　　You are (　　　)(　　　)(　　　)(　　　).
Miriam:　I know those things are absurd but (　　　)(　　　)(　　　) (　　　). They're so mysterious and attractive.

VI MORE ABOUT AMERICAN HEALTH ISSUES

> **アメリカにおける医師と病院の関係　Health Practitioners in America**
>
> 　日本では、医師と病院の関係は雇用関係で結ばれている。しかし、アメリカでは、医師は「ソロ・プラクティショナー (solo practitioner)」や「プライベート・プラクティショナー (private practitioner)」と呼ばれ、個人開業医として、各自のクリニックで患者を診察し、日本のように病院の外来で患者を治療することは基本的には行わない。クリニックも、日本のように一人で診察する場合もあるが、その多くが、3人以上の医師が共同で診療を行う「グループ・プラクティス」である。自分のクリニックでは実施できない検査（MRIなど）や手術、それに伴う入院治療は、自分の契約している病院へ出向いて、病院の施設を利用して、自分の患者の治療を行う。すなわち患者も、医師を選ぶのに際し、医師とクリニックの評判ばかりでなく、グループ診療でのほかの医師について、さらに、その医師が契約を結んでいる病院がどこにあり、どういう施設を備えている病院であるかも重要な要因となる。
>
> 　医師が病院との施設利用契約やグループ・プラクティス組織と雇用契約を結ぶ場合、病院やグループ・プラクティス組織は、医師の実績と経験を調査するため、厳密な書類審査や面接を要求する。そして病院もまた、優秀な医師と契約を結ぶために、最新の医療設備や質の高いパラメディカル・スタッフを提供するなどの努力を図っている。

VII YOUR OPINIONS

次の英語の質問に対し、英語または日本語で答えてみましょう。後で、グループで話し合ってみるのも良いでしょう。

Q. Miriam was only the second patient from the group described here to have truly benefited from the L-dopa treatment. Given that the patients who did not ultimately benefit from the therapy actually suffered quite marked side-effects from the drug treatment, do you think the L-dopa approach was worthwhile?

Epilogue

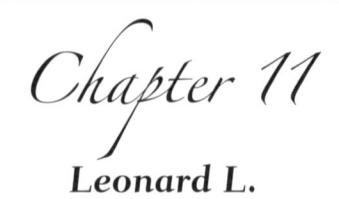

Chapter 11
Leonard L.

　レナードは、いったんは L-dopa による治療をあきらめていましたが、1974 〜 1980 年に再びその服用を試みます。結果はどうなるのでしょうか。レナードは、1969 年に経験した目覚めを再び体験することができるのでしょうか。

I PRE-READING

Parkinson's disease（パーキンソン病）

How much do you know about Parkinson's disease (PD)? Decide if the statements below are T (true) or F (False).

(1) (　) The exact cause of PD is unknown.
(2) (　) Although PD may appear in younger patients, it usually affects middle-aged people.
(3) (　) Genetic predisposition definitely does not play a role in the development of PD.
(4) (　) Some social, economic, and geographical factors very clearly play a role in the development of PD.
(5) (　) Parkinson's disease is chronic (persists over a long period of time), and progressive.

II VOCABULARY & IDIOMATIC EXPRESSIONS

The following terms are used in the story below. Match each of the following words or phrases (①-⑥) with the correct definitions (meaning 'in context') from the box below (a-f). Also choose the appropriate Japanese translation (ア-カ) for each term.

下の語（句）は、すべて **STORY** に出てくるものです。それぞれの英語の説明として、ふさわしいものを a〜f の中から選びなさい。さらにその日本語の意味として、最もふさわしいものをア〜カの中から選びなさい。

① mirror　　　　　(　)(　)　　② drastic　　　(　)(　)
③ rage　　　　　　(　)(　)　　④ inexplicably (　)(　)
⑤ baseline state (　)(　)　　⑥ composed　　(　)(　)

76

a) that cannot be explained or accounted for
b) calm, rather than upset or angry
c) likely to have a strong or far-reaching effect; radical and extreme
d) to feel very angry about something and show it in the way one behaves or speaks
e) standard conditions and facts for a point of comparison, especially in medicine or science
f) to be very similar to something or to be a copy of something

ア　思い切った、抜本的な　　　　イ　酷似している　　ウ　激怒する
エ　不可解にも、説明できないほどに　オ　平静な、静かな　カ　基準(基礎)の状態

III COMPREHENSION

The following story will help you understand what happened to Leonard after 1972. Please read and answer the true or false questions below.

次の英文を読んで、正しいものにはT、間違っているものにはFをつけましょう。

STORY

After the final trial of amantadine in March 1972, Leonard decided that he 'had had it with drugs' and told Dr. Sacks that he could 'keep his L-dopa.' He then reverted back to his pre-L-dopa status. Despite claiming that he had accepted his fate, he continued to hope that perhaps he could change his luck and try L-dopa again. Leonard finally did decide to give it another try. This happened after he became particularly encouraged by the unexpected and amazing response to L-dopa of another post-encephalitic (PE) patient, Gertie C., when she was put back on the drug after a gap of four years.

Sadly, Leonard experienced the same intense sensitivity to L-dopa in September 1974 as he had in September 1969. Leonard then asked to be put on amantadine and he underwent numerous amantadine trials from 1974 to 1980, but the results mirrored those of 1969 to 1972. At first, Leonard improved but then the results became less and less favorable, until even his 'baseline' state became worse and worse so that without medication he was unable to function.

Until 1977, Leonard had retained a state of good general health. After that, due to the effects of his medication and because of numerous cost-cutting measures which resulted in a drastic reduction of daily care, Leonard suffered weight loss, choked on his food, had urinary infections, and developed bedsores. By 1978, everyone including Leonard realized that he was a very ill man, but Leonard 'raged' to continue living. By 1980, however, he questioned whether it was worth living or not as he used his letter board to spell out, "It's pain and pus, pus and pain. Not worth living. Not a life."

By the end of 1980, amantadine was producing only negative effects. Therefore, L-dopa was given to Leonard because of concerns that his life was at stake. Inexplicably, the L-dopa worked for the first time in twelve years—Leonard became stronger and his strong voice returned. However, Leonard was very unhappy to be reawakened at a time when his body was in such a bad state and he pleaded to be allowed to 'die in peace.'

Dr. Sacks agreed to honor Leonard's wishes and immediately stopped the L-dopa and Leonard reverted to his former silence. Leonard seemed very composed and when his death came it was gentle and a release from his life of suffering.

Notes

2 **have it with**「〜に別れを告げる」　3 **pre-L-dopa status**「L-dopa 以前の状態」　7 **amazing**「驚嘆すべき」　10 **the same intense sensitivity to**「〜に対し同様な激しい敏感さ」　12 **undergo**「受ける」　12 **numerous**「非常に多くの」　14 **favorable**「良好な」　17 **retain**「保っている」　17 **state of good general health**「全体的に良い健康状態」　18-**cost-cutting measure**「費用を削減する手段」　19 **daily care**「日常の世話」　20 **urinary infection**「泌尿器感染症」　21 **bedsore**「床ずれ」　24 **pus**「うみ、膿汁」　28 **at stake**「危機に瀕して」　31 **plead**「〜を懇願する」　32 **honor**「〜を尊重する」

True or False Questions

1. (　) Leonard never tried the L-dopa treatment again after 1972.
2. (　) Because the amantadine treatment worked better than the L-dopa treatment, Leonard continued to take it and was able to lead an active life until he died.
3. (　) Leonard decided to try L-dopa again after he heard that Gertie had shown an excellent response when she was put back on L-dopa after a four year interval.
4. (　) Due to the effects of his medication and staff reductions which resulted in a much lower level of care-giving, Leonard's condition worsened after 1977.
5. (　) After 1980, even though Leonard was really sick and weak, he had a strong will to live.

IV USEFUL EXPRESSIONS

The following sentences were used in Dr. Sacks' original book. Use the hints below to help you to accurately translate the sentences into Japanese.

次の英文は、すべてサックス博士の小説 *Awakenings* に出てくるものです。それぞれの語（句）の注を参考に、日本語に訳してみましょう。

1. He <u>consulted with</u> his mother—most decisions were made together—and now asked that amantadine be tried: "I can <u>hardly be worse</u>," he tapped; "it had some use before."

   _____

   _____

   consult with ～「～に相談する」　**hardly be worse**「ほとんど悪くはならない」

2. "<u>Do you suppose</u>," he whispered, "that <u>my receptors are dying off</u>? I don't know whether medication cures them or kills them."

   _____

   _____

   do you suppose ～?「あなたは～と思いますか」　**one's receptors are dying off**「～の（薬の）受容体は次々と死んでいっている」

3. But his <u>bedsores</u> got deeper and deeper, causing <u>ceaseless pain</u>, fever, and <u>sepsis</u>, and <u>draining</u> him of <u>vitally needed protein</u>.

   _____

   _____

   bedsore(s)「床ずれ」　**ceaseless pain**「絶え間のない痛み」　**sepsis**「敗血症」　**drain**「流しだす」　**vitally needed protein**「（生命にかかわるほど）極めて必要なたんぱく質」

4. By the end of 1980, amantadine <u>had wholly ceased</u> to 'work'—or, rather, produced only <u>pathological effects</u>. Early in 1981, therefore, <u>after searching discussion</u>, feeling that life was <u>at stake</u>, and it had to be used, we tried him once again on L-dopa.

   _____

79

have wholly ceased「完全に止まった」   **pathological effect(s)**「病的な効力・効果」   **after searching discussion**「議論を重ねた後」   **at stake**「危機に瀕して」

5. I had no idea what went on inside him—but I felt he was conscious, though <u>turned to</u> <u>Last Things</u>.

turn to ~「~に取り掛かる」   **Last Things**「死（の準備）」

V LISTENING FOCUS   CD 23
Please listen to the passage and fill in the blanks with words or expressions.

次の会話を聞いて、空欄の英語を聞き取ってみましょう。

Dialog 11
After Leonard's death, Dr. Sacks wrote a letter of condolence to Leonard's mother. In this letter, Dr. Sacks explained the effect that Leonard had had on his life.

What I felt in 1966 I felt more strongly every year—what a remarkable man Leonard was. What courage and humor he showed, in the face of an almost life-long (-   )(   ). I tried to (   )(   )(   ) this feeling when I wrote of him in *Awakenings* … but was conscious of how inadequate and partial this was.

I have never had a patient who taught me so much—not simply about parkinsonism, but what it means to be a human being, who survives, and fully, (   )(   )(   )(   ) such affliction and such (   )(   ). Now Leonard has gone, there will be a (   ) (   ) and a great grief.

Ⅵ MORE ABOUT AMERICAN HEALTH ISSUES

安楽死　Euthanasia

　安楽死の定義は、苦しい生、意味のない生から患者を解放するという目的で、意図的になされた死、またはその目的を達成するために行われる「死なせる」行為のことである。古代ギリシャ・ローマ時代の人々は、人間は理性的な存在であり、無意味と思われる生に対しては、自殺や他人の帮助による死を選ぶこともあると考えられてきた。しかしキリスト教の影響が強くなると、聖書によって人為的な死は厳しく戒められるようになり、5世紀以後ヨーロッパでは、自殺は宗教上の罪となった。安楽死も自殺幇助であり、自殺と同様に罪であると考えられた。これに対し、17世紀イギリスのフランシス・ベーコンは、不治の病の場合は尊厳死を認めるトマス・モアの考えを引き継ぎ、安楽死という言葉(euthanasie)を使用した。1930年代にはヨーロッパで安楽死の是非についての討論が始まり、現在に至っている。

　安楽死は大別すると次の二つに分けられる。

　<u>積極的安楽死</u>　薬物を投与するなど積極的方法で死期を早めること。医療の範疇で行われる自殺幇助という意味合いで、社会からの心理的抵抗が大きい。また、日本を含む多くの国では刑事犯罪として扱われる。

　<u>消極的安楽死</u>　延命治療を行わないで死に至らせること。尊厳死を保つ意味からも合法的で社会的に認知されており、実際の医療現場でも行われる。(**Do not resuscitate〔DNR〕**：人工蘇生をするべからず)

　現在、積極的安楽死を認めている事例としては、国別ではスイスが1942年にこれを認めたのをはじめとし、オランダ(2001年)、ベルギー(2002年)、ルクセンブルク(2008年)で「安楽死法」が可決され、フランス(2005年)では「尊厳死法」が可決された。その他、アメリカでは、オレゴン州で1994年「尊厳死法(Death with Dignity Act)」が成立し、ワシントン州(2009年)、モンタナ州(2009年)、バーモント州(2013年)、ニューメキシコ州(2014年)、カリフォルニア州(2015年)がこれに続いている。

　日本では、これに関わる事件として、名古屋安楽死事件(昭和37年12月22日判決)と、東海大学安楽死事件がある。名古屋安楽死事件は家族内で起こった事件であるが、東海大学安楽死事件は、病院に入院していた末期がん症状の患者に塩化カリウムを投与して、患者を死に至らしめたとして、担当の内科医であった大学助手が殺人罪に問われた。これは日本においての刑事裁判で医師による安楽死の正当性が問われた初めての事件であった。この事件で横浜地方裁判所(平成7年3月28日判決)は、被告人を有罪(懲役2年執行猶予2年)とした。このとき、医師による積極的安楽死として、以下の許容されるための4要件を出した。すなわち、1.患者が絶えがたい激しい肉体的苦痛で苦しんでいること　2.患者の死が避けられず、その死期が迫っていること　3.患者の肉体的苦痛を除去・緩和するための方法を尽くし、他に代替手段がないこと　4.生命の短縮を承諾する患者の明示の意思表示があることを必要とする。

VII YOUR OPINIONS

次の英語の質問に対し、英語または日本語で答えてみましょう。後で、グループで話し合ってみるのも良いでしょう。

Q. The budget cuts in the late 1970's were indirectly responsible for Leonard's rapid deterioration. Special care facilities, which focus mostly on a relatively small subset of society, are often severely impacted by staffing shortages. Do you think that some of these problems can be addressed by more closely involving family members and the community in the care of these patients? It can be useful to examine this in the context of rapidly aging societies, which will face many of the same types of issues concerning extended special care.

_____
_____
_____
_____

VIII MEDICAL ENGLISH ENHANCER（英語で調べてみよう）

Complete a short (6-7 sentences) summary of the following medical term(s). Use English references as your source material.

アメリカや日本以外の国の看護師（nurse）について、その働き、役割、資格などを英語の文献で調べ、それを7行程度の英文でまとめてみましょう。それを参考に日本と比較してみましょう。

_____
_____
_____
_____
_____
_____

Chapter 12
Rose R. and Hester Y.

　ローズは、L-dopa によって目覚めた後も、眠りに入った1926年から自分を解き放つことができずにいました。その後、彼女は現実を受け入れることができたのでしょうか。一方、ヘスターは強い意志によって L-dopa の副作用と闘い、自分を保つことができていましたが、その後の生活はどのようなものだったのでしょうか。

Ⅰ PRE-READING
Clinical Trials（治験）

The following is about the drug development process in the US. Please answer the questions below.

The process of discovering and developing safe and effective new medicines is long, difficult, and expensive. (　1　) Preclinical Testing, Investigational New Drug Application (IND), Clinical Testing, New Drug Application (NDA), and Approval.

Ⅰ　以下の英語の質問の答えとして、最も適切なものを①〜④の中から選びなさい。
(Q1) Which of the following would be the BEST substitute for (　1　)?
　① To earn enormous profits, the following steps are used:
　② The entire drug development process can be summarized as follows:
　③ Only one of the following steps is needed to approve every drug :
　④ The approval process for both drugs and health supplements include the following steps:

Ⅱ　本文中の下線の用語について、日本語の意味として、最もふさわしいものを①から⑤の中から選びなさい。
1. Clinical Testing（　　）　　　　2. Preclinical Testing（　　）
3. Investigational New Drug Application (IND)（　　）
4. New Drug Application (NDA)（　　）　5. Approval（　　）

① 前臨床試験　② 臨床試験　③ 新薬（承認）申請
④ 承認　　　　⑤ 研究用新薬申請

II VOCABULARY & IDIOMATIC EXPRESSIONS

The following terms are used in the story below. Match each of the following words or phrases (①–⑥) with the correct definitions (meaning 'in context') from the box below (a–f). Also choose the appropriate Japanese translation (ア–カ) for each term.

下の語（句）は、すべて **STORY** に出てくるものです。それぞれの英語の説明として、ふさわしいものを a～f の中から選びなさい。さらにその日本語の意味として、最もふさわしいものをア～カの中から選びなさい。

① forge　　　　（　）（　）　　② commence　（　）（　）
③ uncanny　　（　）（　）　　④ settle down　（　）（　）
⑤ prediction　（　）（　）　　⑥ curtail　　　（　）（　）

> a) very strange and difficult to explain
> b) a statement that says what one thinks will happen; the act of making such a statement
> c) to stop behaving in an excited way
> d) to begin or to start something
> e) to develop a strong bond or link with someone else
> f) reduce in extent or quantity

ア　予言　　　　　　　　イ　（友好などを）結ぶ　　ウ　異常な
エ　開始する、着手する　オ　静まる、安定する　　　カ　縮小する、削減する

III COMPREHENSION

The following story will help you understand what happened to Rose and Hester after 1972. Please read and answer the true or false questions below.

次の英文を読んで、正しいものには T、間違っているものには F をつけましょう。

STORY — CD 24

　　Dr. Sacks had always regarded Rose's case as the most uncanny among his post-encephalitic (PE) patients, even before he commenced the L-dopa treatment. Rose had responded positively and strikingly to L-dopa only once, back in the summer of 1969. After that, Rose's life was as empty as the years before that single eventful period. She was always somewhat helped by L-dopa but never to the same extent as her dramatic improvement in 1969. She suffered severe oculogyric crises and kept saying, "I'm going to die, I'm going to die." Unfortunately, in June 1979, her prediction came true as she choked to death on a chicken bone. Her life had been one of great illness which most people would have had trouble imagining, much less experiencing.

Hester experienced a very unique, explosive reaction to the L-dopa treatment. Unlike other patients who experienced initial violent reactions and settled down or had positive reactions with lessening effects, Hester's reactions remained extremely violent. Importantly, Hester was able to put herself 'above' these reactions, which might have been fatal in other patients.

In 1981, Hester was still on L-dopa, and still suffered explosive reactions, but she refused to curtail her personal activities such as bingo, gardening, poetry readings and excursions. She did lose her ability to walk independently but like many patients at Mount Carmel, she forged a close relationship with another patient. This patient not only tended to Hester's more practical needs, such as pushing her wheelchair around the hospital, but she also understood what Hester was thinking and feeling. Despite losing her mobility, her disease was basically at a standstill. Interestingly, Dr Sacks observed that this was the case with most of his PE patients, and that this was in stark contrast with ordinary Parkinson's disease patients whose conditions always seemed to go downhill, even if on a slow and progressive course.

From May 17, 1969, when she exploded in response to L-dopa, Hester began to have a life. Before that, she had been, for all intents and purposes, 'asleep.' By 1982, Hester had been awake for twelve and a half years, and at the time he wrote *Awakenings*, Dr. Sacks saw no reason why she should not continue to do so for the rest of her life.

Notes

3 **strikingly**「顕著に、際立って」　5 **single eventful period**「一度きりの多事多端な時期」　7 **dramatic improvement**「劇的な改善」　7 **oculogyric crisis**「注視痙攣」　12 **explosive reaction**「激しい反応」　20 **excursion**「小旅行」　25 **at a standstill**「足踏み状態、休止状態」　27 **in stark contrast with**「〜と全く対照的に」　28 **go downhill**「悪化する」　29 **progressive course**「進行性の経過」　31-**for all intents and purposes**「どの点から見ても、大筋で」

True or False Questions

1. (　) Rose was happy and comfortable when she died because after the L-dopa treatment, she had recovered and lived a normal life.
2. (　) Rose was administered L-dopa only once during her stay at Mount Carmel.
3. (　) The majority of patients with Parkinson's disease had positive results with L-dopa treatment.
4. (　) Hester was one of the long-term L-dopa success stories at Mount Carmel.
5. (　) Hester had a close friend at Mount Carmel who supported her both mentally and physically.

IV USEFUL EXPRESSIONS

The following sentences were used in Dr. Sacks' original book. Use the hints below to help you to accurately translate the sentences into Japanese.

次の英文は、すべてサックス博士の小説 ***Awakenings*** に出てくるものです。それぞれの語（句）の注を参考に、日本語に訳してみましょう。

1. She had been <u>inconceivably, inaccessibly, and incommunicably ill</u> since the <u>nightmare-night</u> she became ill, in 1926.

   inconceivably, inaccessibly and incommunicably ill「考えられないほど（深く）、近づき難いほど、そして、意思疎通を取ることもできないほど（重く）病気にかかっている」　**nightmare-night**「悪夢を見た夜」

2. I see now that <u>this is the case with</u> most of our post-encephalitic patients, and <u>it distinguishes them absolutely from</u> patients with ordinary Parkinson's disease, who have to face a <u>steadily downhill</u> if <u>slow and progressive, course</u>.

   this is the case with ～「これが～の症例」　**it distinguishes ～ absolutely from…**「それは～を明確に…と区別する」　**steadily downhill**「着実な下り坂」　**slow and progressive, course**「ゆっくりとした進行性の経過」

3. There are a number of these friendships at Mount Carmel, which shine with <u>a singular moral radiance</u> in the tragic, and sometimes <u>hellish</u>, darkness of the place.

_____

_____

a singular moral radiance「唯一の精神的な輝き」 **hellish**「地獄のような」

4. The matter, clearly is <u>extraordinarily complex</u>—Hester has <u>a great deal going against</u> her, and <u>a great deal for</u> her.

_____

_____

extraordinarily complex「驚くほど複雑」 **a great deal going against** ～「～に逆らう多くの力」 **a great deal for** ～「～を支える多くの力」

Ⅴ LISTENING FOCUS　　　　　　　　　　　　　　　　　CD 25

Please listen to Chapter 12-Dialog 12 (the text is reproduced below) and fill in the blanks with appropriate words, expressions, or phrases.

次の会話を聞いて、空欄の英語を聞き取ってみましょう。

Dialog 12

Even though Hester was ultimately one of the most successful cases for the L-dopa treatment, she did, at one point, ask for the treatments to be stopped, because of the great changes they were having on her.

Hester: Dr. Sacks, please stop the L-dopa. It's (　　　) (　　　) (　　　) (　　　).
Dr. Sacks: I understand what you mean, but you have improved so much and before, you didn't even want me to lower your dosage.
Hester: I know, but (　　　) (　　　) (　　　) (　　　) (　　　).
Dr. Sacks: I can do that.
Hester: Good, I need to (　　　) (　　　) and (　　　) (　　　) (　　　).

Ⅵ MORE ABOUT AMERICAN HEALTH ISSUES

アメリカの医療保険制度 (American Health Insurance System)

　アメリカの医療保険制度は、公的医療保険と民間医療保健から成り立っている。公的医療保険は、高齢者、低所得者、軍人などの約34％の人々が加入しており、それ以外の一般国民は、個人や企業を通して、民間医療保険を利用している。公的医療保険は、老人医療保険、低所得者医療保険、軍人医療保険、子供医療保険など、6種類の保険制度であるが、民間医療保険はその種類も多種多様である。民間医療保険はさまざまな契約によって運営されており、保険会社、医療機関、被保険者の間でその手続きも多く、間違いも生じやすいのが現状である。

　日本とアメリカの保険制度の大きな違いは、日本人が国民健康保険という公的保険でほぼカバーされているのに対し、アメリカ人の多くは民間の保険を利用している点である。民間の保険とは、日本の民間の保険とほぼ同じ役割を担っており、既往歴でカバーされない手術や治療費が生じることにより、個人の負担する医療費の高くなったり、雇用主が加入している保険適応度などによって、負担額が増えたりするなどの違いがある。こうした中、2014年オバマ大統領が国民皆保険制度である「オバマケア」を施行した。しかしながら、施行当初より問題が続出し、現在もまだ先が見えない状況にある。

Ⅶ YOUR OPINIONS

次の英語の質問に対し、英語または日本語で答えてみましょう。後で、グループで話し合ってみるのも良いでしょう。

Q. Parkinson's disease patients suffer problems with brain dopamine levels. Interestingly, the L-dopa treatment was more successful therapeutically for Dr. Sacks' PE patients than for Parkinson's disease patients. Does this surprise you?

Ⅷ MEDICAL ENGLISH ENHANCER（英語で調べてみよう）

Complete a short (6-7 sentences) summary of the following medical term(s). Use English references as your source material.

アメリカや日本以外の国の理学療法士（physical therapist: PT）または作業療法士（occupational therapist: OT）のうち興味のあるものを1つ選び、その働き、役割、資格などを英語の文献で調べ、それを8行程度の英文でまとめてみましょう。それを参考に日本と比較してみましょう。

Chapter 13

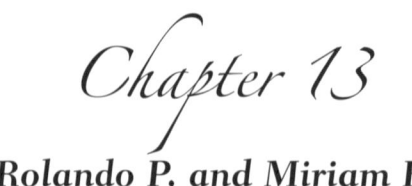

Rolando P. and Miriam H.

　ロランドは、L-dopa の投与後も自分の状態に悲観的でしたが、果たして平穏な生活が送れるようになったのでしょうか。また、ミリアムのその後の経過は、どのようなものだったのでしょう。

I PRE-READING

Neurological Infections（神経系感染症）

Viruses and microorganisms sometimes invade the body, infecting various organs and causing everything from mild disturbances to serious problems. Bacterial organisms are often to blame, but animal parasites and fungi can also cause infection. Neurological infections occur when these viruses and organisms invade the nervous system.

Symptoms of Infection:
Pain, swelling, redness, impaired function and fever are all characteristics of an infection. There may also be heat at the site of the infected area. In the case of some viral infections, drowsiness, confusion and convulsions may occur.

Types of Neurological Infections:
The three diseases listed below are the most common neurological infections. Please match each disease with the correct corresponding definition for the condition. Also, please choose the appropriate Japanese translation（ア－カ）for each term.

① encephalitis（　　）（　　）　　② meningitis（　　）（　　）
③ HIV（　　）（　　）

a) a viral infection that causes AIDS and gradually destroys the body's immune system
b) an inflammation of the membranes that cover the brain and spinal cord, which can be caused by either bacteria or virus
c) an inflammation of the brain, which can be caused by either bacteria or virus.

ア．髄膜炎　　　イ．ヒト免疫不全ウイルス　　　ウ．脳炎

Source: Neurological Infections ¦ University of Maryland Medical Centerhttp://umm.edu/programs/neurosciences/services/neurological-infections#ixzz3glu0h7MD University of Maryland Medical Center

II VOCABULARY & IDIOMATIC EXPRESSIONS

The following terms are used in the story below. Match each of the following words or phrases (①–⑥) with the correct definitions (meaning 'in context') from the box below (a–f). Also choose the appropriate Japanese translation (ア–カ) for each term.

下の語（句）は、すべて **STORY** に出てくるものです。それぞれの英語の説明として、ふさわしいものをa～fの中から選びなさい。さらにその日本語の意味として、最もふさわしいものをア～カの中から選びなさい。

① force O to ~　　　　（　）（　）　　② trigger　　　　　　　（　）（　）
③ be compounded by （　）（　）　　④ be resentful about （　）（　）
⑤ sink into　　　　　　（　）（　）　　⑥ settle into　　　　　　（　）（　）

> a) to move gradually into a negative state of emotion
> b) to make a difficult situation worse by adding more problems
> c) to make someone do something they do not want to do
> d) feeling angry and upset about something that you think is unfair
> e) to make a final choice on one's condition or environment
> f) to cause an event or situation to happen

ア　～に沈みこむ　　　　　　　　　　イ　引き金を引く、きっかけとなる
ウ　～を嫌がっている、怒っている　　エ　余儀なくOに～させる
オ　（～の状態に）落ち着く　　　　　カ　度合いを強める、輪をかける

III COMPREHENSION

The following story will help you understand what happened to Rolando and Miriam after 1972. Please read and answer the true or false questions below.

次の英文を読んで、正しいものにはT、間違っているものにはFをつけましょう。

STORY

Rolando had a devoted mother. She was a regular visitor every Sunday until severe arthritis in the summer of 1972 forced her to curtail her visits. This change in events triggered, in Rolando, a dramatic negative emotional reaction which resulted in a two month period of depression, rage, and grief, during which he lost twenty pounds. Fate intervened in the form of a new physiotherapist at Mount Carmel whose professional gifts combined with a warm and loving nature led Rolando to develop an intimate 'anaclitic' relationship with her. This therapist's devotion was complete and she often gave up her personal time on weekends and evenings to be with Rolando. He came to rely on her as he had on his mother. In this environment, Rolando became calmer and better-humored. Not only that, he gained weight and he could sleep well. Things seemed set to continue in a positive way.

Unfortunately, this did not last. In February 1973, this beloved physiotherapist was cut from the staff because of severe budget restraints. This event sent Rolando's health into a tailspin. By the middle of February, he was manifesting signs of a severe mental breakdown, compounded by grief, depression, terror, and rage. Towards the end of February he had settled into a death-like apathy. It was clear that he had lost the will to live and one day simply refused to have his lab test, "Can't you see I'm dying of grief? Please let me die in peace!" he yelled. Just four days later, he died in his sleep.

In the end, it was Miriam who did the best—she not only had the fullest life but also suffered the least complications. She needed to be kept on a substantial dose of L-dopa which was acceptable as she had no serious side-effects which would have warranted any reduction. Miriam had spent a total of fifty years at Mount Carmel. Thanks to L-dopa, from 1972 her life had been free from complications, in marked contrast to the previous thirty-seven years spent sinking into a hopeless state. At sixty-five years of age, she looked much younger than her years, possessed a keen intellect and was full of energy and life.

Like many other patients who had benefited from L-dopa Miriam wished that L-dopa had arrived earlier. But she was not resentful about it and looked forward with optimism to her future.

Notes

2 **arthritis**「関節炎」　5 **intervene**「入る、現われる」　6-**professional gift**「職業的な資質」　8 **intimate**「親しい」　8 **'anaclitic' relationship**「母親依存性の関係」　11-**good-humored**「機嫌の良い、快活な」　15 **be cut from**「～から解雇される」　15-**budget restraint(s)**「経費抑制」　16 **tailspin**「きりもみ降下」　17 **manifest**「(兆候などが)現われる」　17 **mental breakdown**「神経衰弱」　18 **terror**「恐怖」　19 **apathy**「無関

心」　25 **substantial**「十分な」　26 **warrant**「正当化する、当然のことである」
26 **reduction**「減少」　30 **possess**「（人が才能などを）持つ」　34 **optimism**「楽観主義」

True or False Questions

1. (　) After Rolando recovered from the emotional crisis due to the loss of his mother, he was saved by one physiotherapist who took care of him like his mother had done.
2. (　) Rolando died in unhappy circumstances.
3. (　) Miriam's condition deteriorated after 1980 because L-dopa didn't work for her any more.
4. (　) At Mount Carmel, cost cuts resulted in the dismissal of some staff in 1973.
5. (　) It can be said that Miriam's life was saved by the L-dopa treatment.

IV USEFUL EXPRESSIONS

The following sentences were used in Dr. Sacks' original book. Use the hints below to help you to accurately translate the sentences into Japanese.

次の英文は、すべてサックス博士の小説 *Awakenings* に出てくるものです。それぞれの語（句）の注を参考に、日本語に訳してみましょう。

1. Under this benign and healing influence, Rolando's wound began to heal over—he became calmer and better-humored, gained weight, and slept well.

   _____

   _____

   benign「優しい、慈悲深い」　**heal over**「（病気や傷などが）治る、回復する」
   better-humored (good-humored)「陽気な、機嫌の良い」

2. Unfortunately, at the start of February, his beloved physiotherapist was dismissed from her job (along with almost a third of the hospital staff) as a result of economies dictated by the recent federal budget.

   _____

   _____

   be dismissed from ~「~から解雇される」　**along with ~**「~と伴に」　**economies dictated by ~**「~によって命じられた節減」　**federal budget**「政府の予算」

3. 'No use crying over spilt milk....' One has to **carry on**—life goes on regardless …

_____

_____

   'No use crying over spilt milk'「覆水盆に返らず」　**life goes on regardless**「人生はお構いなく続く」

4. Roland seemed determined to bear with his loss and live on'regardless'; but at a deeper level, so it seemed to me, he had sustained a wound from which he would not recover.

_____

_____

   determine to bear with ~「~に耐える決心をする」　**sustain a wound**「傷を負う」

5. It is clear, from both clinical observation and EEG, that Miriam is not only 'awakened,' but somewhat 'turned on' by L-dopa.

_____

_____

   clinical observation「臨床的な観察」　**be 'turned on'**「刺激を受ける」

V LISTENING FOCUS　　　　　　　　　　　　　　　CD 27

Please listen to Chapter 13-Dialog 13 (the text is reproduced below) and fill in the blanks with appropriate words, expressions, or phrases.

次の会話を聞いて、空欄の英語を聞き取ってみましょう。

Dialog 13

After Rolando's mother stopped coming due to her arthritis and advanced age, and his surrogate mother, an occupational therapist, was dismissed as a result of budget cuts, Rolando alternated between acceptance of his being alone and intense grief. One day, he was scheduled to have tests.

Lab technician(L.T):　Good Morning, Rolando. How are you this morning?
　　　　　　　　　　(　　　)(　　　)(　　　)(　　　), please.
Rolando:　　　　　　Here you are. What are you doing? Can't you (　　　)
　　　　　　　　　　(　　　)(　　　)?

L.T:	We only want to do a few tests, Rolando. It will (　　　) (　　　) a (　　　).
Rolando:	First my mother stopped coming and now the hospital has taken away the only other person who understood me. You all betrayed me.
L.T:	It couldn't be helped, we are all suffering because of the cuts.
Rolando:	(　　　)(　　　)(　　　). She's a faithless… bitch. I hate her.
L.T:	You (　　　)(　　　)(　　　) Rolando.
Rolando:	Oh. Leave me alone. Don't you (　　　)(　　　)(　　　)(　　　) in your head? Can't you see I'm dying of grief.

VI MORE ABOUT AMERICAN HEALTH ISSUES

Americans with Disabilities Act；ADA（アメリカ障害者法）とは

　1990年7月、アメリカでは、身体的・精神的な障害を理由とした差別を禁止した「アメリカ障害者法」(Americans with Disabilities Act；ADA) が制定された。これは、アメリカに住み障害を持つ人たちに、社会に参加する権利を保障し、そのために必要なホテル・レストラン・劇場・スポーツ施設・官庁などの公共施設や商業施設、飛行場・地下鉄・バスなどの交通機関を、障害の程度に関わらずに利用できるように整備することを義務づけている。また、障害を理由に雇用や教育を差別することも禁じている。電話会社に対しては、耳の不自由な人や言語の不自由な人々に向けての特別サービスを提供するように、義務化している。ADA法には建築の最低基準を定めたADAアクセシビリティ・スタンダードがあり、例えば、車椅子利用に必要な通路幅、エレベータの開閉スピード、階段の手すりの形状などが細かく定められている。

　現在、ADA法の対象となるアメリカ人は、約4300万人と推定されており、人口全体の18％にもなる。ADA法の施行は社会に大きな変化をもたらし、障害者への理解と対応が大きく変わることになった。

VII YOUR OPINIONS

次の英語の質問に対し、英語または日本語で答えてみましょう。後で、グループで話し合ってみるのも良いでしょう。

Q. Miriam and Rolando offer contrasting cases—Miriam survived her ordeal whereas Rolando succumbed to his circumstances. Can you think of any special factors that might explain this contradiction?

_____
_____
_____
_____

Ⅷ MEDICAL ENGLISH ENHANCER（英語で調べてみよう）

Complete a short (6-7 sentences) summary of the following medical term(s). Use English references as your source material.

アメリカや日本以外の国の言語聴覚士（speech-language pathologist: SLP）または視能訓練士（orthoptist: ORT）のうち興味のあるものを1つ選び、それぞれの働き、役割、資格などを英語の文献で調べ、それを8行程度の英文でまとめてみましょう。それを参考に日本と比較してみましょう。

Chapter 14
The Movie AWAKENINGS

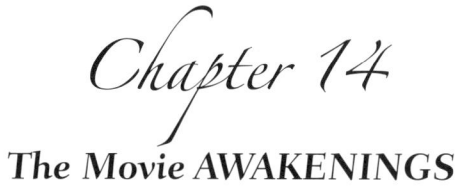

　ロバート・デ・ニーロが迫真の演技で迫る、邦題『レナードの朝』は、原作者のオリバー・サックス博士が製作に加わったことでも知られています。そのハリウッド映画は、しかしながら、細部に及んで原作と相違点があります。ここでは、それらの違いについて考えることで、さらに原作を深く読んでいきましょう。

Ⅰ VOCABULARY & IDIOMATIC EXPRESSIONS

The following terms are used in the story below. Match each of the following words or phrases (①−⑥) with the correct definitions (meaning 'in context') from the box below (a−f). Also choose the appropriate Japanese translation (ア−カ) for each term.

下の語（句）は、すべて **STORY** に出てくるものです。それぞれの英語の説明として、ふさわしいものをa〜fの中から選びなさい。さらにその日本語の意味として、最もふさわしいものをア〜カの中から選びなさい。

① wonderment 　　（　）（　）　　② progressively 　（　）（　）
③ supervision 　　（　）（　）　　④ recipient 　　　（　）（　）
⑤ apprehensively （　）（　）　　⑥ fulfillment 　　（　）（　）

---
a) a person who receives something
b) worried or frightened that something unpleasant may happen
c) a feeling of being satisfied and happy
d) the act of observing and directing someone or something
e) a feeling of pleasant surprise or wonder
f) steadily and continuously

ア　次第に　　　　　　　　　イ　管理　　　　　　　ウ　好奇心
エ　受領者、レシピエント　　オ　満足感、達成感　　カ　懸念して、おずおずと

II COMPREHENSION

The following story will help you understand what happened in the movie AWAKENINGS. Please read and answer the true or false questions below.

次の英文を読んで、正しいものには T、間違っているものには F をつけましょう。

STORY

The movie starts by showing Dr. Malcolm Sayer applying for a job, in 1969, at the chronic-care hospital in the New York Bronx. Dr. Sayer is apparently very shy and since he was previously actively involved only in research, he has had little experience with patients. This makes it difficult for him to adjust to his new working environment and position as a clinical neurologist dealing mostly with psychiatric and catatonic patients. After an interesting encounter with an elderly catatonic patient named Lucy, Dr. Sayer starts to believe that some of the seemingly hopeless, 'stone-like' post-encephalitis lethargica patients under his care are actually aware and cognizant. One such patient is Leonard, who is especially interesting for Dr. Sayer because of Leonard's special relationship with his devoted mother who visits and talks to him almost everyday.

Later, Dr. Sayer starts to think that the experimental drug L-dopa, which at that time was normally administered in the treatment of Parkinson's disease, might also work for his post-encephalitic (PE) patients. Dr. Sayer finally gets permission from his superiors to administer the drug, but only to one patient.

Dr. Sayer chooses Leonard as the first L-dopa recipient. Leonard responds to L-dopa in an astonishing way—the drug seems to have an explosive, 'awakening' effect. Leonard awakens after being imprisoned in a completely paralyzed state since boyhood. He seems to have a child-like wonderment and passion for every moment of his restored life. Leonard's exuberant embrace of even the simplest of life's pleasures proves to be an important lesson for the timid and cautious Dr. Sayer. Indeed, Dr. Sayer undergoes an 'awakening' of his own as he slowly, with some help from the head nurse, Eleanor, begins to conquer his innate shyness.

Because of his success with Leonard, Dr. Sayer administers L-dopa to the rest of his patients, all of whom then awaken after decades of catatonia and subsequently have to deal with a new life in a new time frame. Leonard meets a young woman, Paula, who regularly visits her sick father at the hospital. Leonard manages to enjoy happy periods with Paula even though their interactions are limited to the hospital area.

Eventually, Leonard begins developing side-effects to the L-dopa, and these negative reactions progressively worsen until he begins to have full body spasms and can hardly move. All of the other patients are forced to apprehensively witness Leonard's deterioration, knowing that the same will eventually happen to them. Dr. Sayer tries to increase the L-dopa dosage for these patients but he finds that he cannot stop the side effects. He is therefore forced to stop the treatment and all the patients eventually revert to their catatonic states.

Although Leonard suffers greatly with the L-dopa treatment, saying that he feels more like a series of tics than an actual human being, he nevertheless puts up with the pain. He also asks Dr. Sayer to film him, in the hope that this might someday help others. Because of his hopeless situation, Leonard has to stop taking L-dopa but first he decides to say good-bye to Paula. This leads to a difficult final encounter with Paula, who finally comes to accept Leonard's fate. Paula learns that Leonard has never danced before. Therefore she manages to give Leonard some peace and sense of fulfillment in a touching scene where Leonard's tics and spasms are somehow muted while they dance.

Leonard returns to his catatonic state soon after, and this is painful for most of the hospital staff. Towards the end of the movie, Dr. Sayer tells a group of hospital grant donors that although the 'awakening' did not last, it was nonetheless very illuminating and reminded all of those involved not to forget to appreciate and *live* life. Despite this seemingly positive outlook, Dr. Sayer still finds himself depressed for failing to keep Leonard 'awake,' but Eleanor tells him that he is a good person and that Leonard considered him to be his best friend. The movie ends with Dr. Sayer, remembering Leonard's advice on *living* every minute of life, asking Eleanor to join him for a cup of coffee.

> **Notes**
> 3 **apparently**「見たところは」　6 **clinical neurologist**「臨床神経科医」　6 **catatonic**「緊張型分裂病」　10 **cognizant**「認識した、知っている」　17 **superior**「上司」　20 **astonishing**「驚くほどの、目覚しい」　21 **being imprisoned**「囚われの身となる、牢入れられる」　22 **paralyzed state**「麻痺をした状態」　24 **exuberant embrace**「喜びにあふれて受け入れること」　27 **conquer**「征服する」　27 **innate**「生来の」　47 **encounter**「出会い」　51 **mute**「消える」　54 **hospital grant donor**「病院補助金寄付者」　55 **illuminating**「啓発する、啓もう的な」

True or False Questions

1. (　) Leonard was the last patient to receive L-dopa from Dr. Sayer at the hospital.
2. (　) Eleanor understood Dr. Sayers's sorrow when Leonard went back to his previous condition.
3. (　) Leonard's mother was a very cold woman who did not care for him very much.
4. (　) Paula gave Leonard some peace toward the end of the movie.
5. (　) Leonard did not like Dr. Sayer because eventually Dr. Sayer could not help him.

III YOUR OPINIONS

次の英文は『レナードの朝』の映画と原作の違いについて述べたものです。英文をよく読んで、後の問いに従って、その違いを考えてみましょう。

　　In the movie, the message is almost the same as that in the novel—that the most life-affirming acts are often simply those that rely on human contact and relationships. However, many details have been changed in the movie, making it a very fictionalized version of the book.

　　The names and characters in the movie are different from those in the book. For example, Oliver Sacks becomes Malcolm Sayer, a caring but somewhat introverted doctor who finds it challenging dealing with people. In some cases, new characters are introduced for dramatic effect, for example, the movie has a head nurse named Eleanor Costello and a young woman, Paula, who regularly visits Leonard. These two protagonists are apparently used to introduce a romantic element within the story.

　　Other plot devices include using fewer characters in the movie than actually existed. Eleanor Costello, in fact, appears to be an amalgam of two real-life nurses, one of whom was Eleanor Gaynor, while the other was called Ellen Costello. What is critical is that these two real-life nurses, along with a number of others, helped Dr. Sacks with his patients. This is also reflected in the movie in the manner in which Eleanor Costello supports Dr. Sayer's work.

Many of the patients in the movie are also represented as having personalities & characteristics that are actually found in multiple real-life patients. Some key elements have been retained, such as Leonard being the first to awaken, and his suffering severe side-effects. However, the situation with the other patients was far more complicated—some were actually able to enjoy remarkable progress after L-dopa treatment whereas others had outcomes similar to that seen with Leonard. In contrast, the movie shows all the patients apprehensively watching Leonard endure the L-dopa side-effects with the knowledge that they would each certainly suffer a similar fate.

Leonard is a difficult character to capture in his entirety, in any medium, and the movie depicts him with some heroic overtones which may or may not reflect some elements of his true nature. One aspect of Leonard's life in which the movie deviated quite dramatically from reality is in Leonard's intellectual and academic achievements—the real Leonard had almost completed a doctorate whereas the movie implied that Leonard received mostly house-based schooling.

One important feature of the storyline, relating to the use and dispensation of L-dopa, is treated in an almost cavalier manner in the movie. Dr. Sayer is shown handling and dealing with L-dopa in a somewhat haphazard way whereas Dr. Sacks was obviously far more cautious in the use of this—at the time—experimental drug. This is again probably a plot device designed to communicate, to laypeople, the uncertainty of this undefined treatment.

Notes

2 **life-affirming act**「生きる勇気を与える行動」　4 **fictionalize**「(事実の記録を) 小説化する」　7 **introvert**「内向的な」　7 **challenging**「骨の折れる、苦しい」　11 **protagonist**「主役」　11 **apparently**「明らかに」　13 **plot device**「筋書きの工夫」　14 **amalgam**「合わせたもの」　20 **represent**「描写する」　21- **multiple real-life patients**「多様な現実の患者たち」　30 **in his entirety**「彼をそっくりそのまま」　30- **in any medium**「どんな媒体でも」　31 **depict**「描く」　33 **deviate**「それる、逸脱する」　38 **dispensation**「調剤、処方」　38 **cavalier manner**「ぞんざいな態度」　40 **haphazard way**「無計画な方法」　42 **communicate**「伝える」

42 **laypeople**「(専門家でない) 素人の人々」　43 **uncertainty**「疑念」　43 **undefined treatment**「不明確な治療」

映画と原作の違いに関する、以下の項目についてまとめなさい。

1. エレノアとポーラの描写について
   _____
   _____
   _____

2. レナード以外の患者の描き方について
   _____
   _____
   _____

3. レナードの描き方について
   _____
   _____
   _____

4. 投薬の仕方とその結果(成功、不成功)の描写について
   _____
   _____
   _____

Ⅳ Oliver Sacks : Personal History and Major Accomplishiments

筆者について

オリバー・サックス

　脳神経科医として、その臨床体験を基にした優れた医学エッセイを数多く発表している。1933年にロンドンで生まれ、オックスフォード大学で医学の学位を取得した後アメリカに渡り、カリフォルニア大学ロサンゼルス校で神経医学の研修医となる。1965年以来、ニューヨークに居住しており、ニューヨーク大学医学部、コロンビア大学医科大学院教授を勤めた。2015年8月30日、ニューヨーク市グリニッジビレッジの自宅にて死去。82歳だった。その9年前に眼球悪性黒色腫により片眼の視力を失った。2015年2月には、肝臓への転移により余命がわずかであることを、メディアを通して告白していた。

　著作には彼が出会った患者について、その治療体験に主眼を置いて描かれたものが多い。サックス博士自身を患者として書いたものもある。多くの場合、患者は完治することはないが、患者の複雑な治療過程が語られ、深い洞察とともに、全体に一貫して流れるヒューマニズムが共通した特徴としてあげられる。

　代表作『レナードの朝』（同名の映画の原作）は、1960年代の終わりに彼が治療した嗜眠性脳炎の患者たちに、当時、パーキンソン病の新薬として開発されたL-ドーパを投与した経験に基づいて書かれたものである。他の著作では、トゥレット障害、片頭痛、知能障害などについて記している。著書は日本語を含む21か国語に翻訳されている。

[代表作品]
　著書『サックス博士の片頭痛大全』（*Migraine* 1970年）『左足をとりもどすまで』（*A Leg to Stand On* 1984年）『妻を帽子とまちがえた男』（*The Man Who Mistook His Wife for a Hat* 1985年）『手話の世界へ』（*Seeing Voices* 1989年）など。

Ⅴ USEFUL MEDICAL TERMINOLOGY

≪ 病気の症状に関する用語 ≫

次の1～12に挙げるものは、病気の症状に関する語句です。それぞれの日本語の意味として最もふさわしいものをア～シの中から選びなさい。

1. inflammation (　　)　　2. diarrhea (　　)　　3. appetite (　　)
4. chill(s) (　　)　　5. vomiting (　　)　　6. headache (　　)
7. shortness of breath (　　)　　8. nausea (　　)　　9. dizziness (　　)
10. insomnia (　　)　　11. hives (　　)　　12. fever (　　)

ア	不眠症	イ	蕁麻疹	ウ	下痢	エ	頭痛
オ	吐き気	カ	炎症	キ	熱	ク	食欲
ケ	めまい	コ	悪寒	サ	息切れ	シ	嘔吐

《 薬の形態に関する用語 》

次の 1 ～ 12 に挙げるものは、薬の形態に関する語句です。それぞれの日本語の意味として最もふさわしいものをア～シの中から選びなさい。

1. pill （　　）
2. tablet （　　）
3. powder （　　）
4. inhalant （　　）
5. ointment （　　）
6. plaster （　　）
7. liquid (solution) （　　）
8. suppository （　　）
9. sublingual tablet （　　）
10. capsule （　　）
11. syrup （　　）
12. emulsion （　　）

ア　舌下錠　　　　イ　丸薬・錠剤　　　ウ　吸入薬　　　エ　錠剤
オ　水薬　　　　　カ　貼り薬　　　　　キ　軟膏　　　　ク　粉薬
ケ　座薬　　　　　コ　シロップ　　　　サ　乳剤　　　　シ　カプセル剤

<参考文献>

小俣和一郎（2005）『精神医学の歴史』第三文明社
河野恵子（2002）『病院の内側から見たアメリカの医療システム』新興医学出版社
　　　　（2006）『病院の外側から見たアメリカの医療システム』新興医学出版社
柳澤信夫（2000）『パーキンソン病―診断と治療』金原出版
Grob, Gerald N.（1944）*The mad among us : A history of the care of American's mentally ill*
　　　　Cambridge : Harvard University Press.
http://www.ninds.nih.gov/disorders/encephalitis_lethargica（2007 年 3 月）
http://www.national mssociety.org/Meds-Amantadine.asp（2006 年 10 月）
http://www.ninds.nih.gov/health_and_medical/pubs/seizures_and epilepsy_htr.htm（2007 年 3 月）
http://www.emedicine.com/neuro/topic664.htm（2006 年 8 月）
http://plato.stanford.edu/entries/euthanasia-voluntary/An overview of voluntary euthanasia
http://www.umm-edu/nervous/perkins.htm（2006 年 8 月）
http://www.fda.gov/cder/regulatory/applications/ndahtm（2007 年 5 月）
http://www.fda.gov/cder/handbook/indhtm（2007 年 2 月）
http://www.ajhp.org/cgi/content/absturct/57/21/129（2007 年 3 月）
http://www.allp.com/drug-dev.htm（2007 年 3 月）
Neurological Infections, University of Maryland Medical Centerhttp://umm.edu/programs/
　　　　neurosciences/services/neurological-infections#ixzz3glu0h7MD University of Maryland
　　　　Medical Center（2015 年 6 月）

　　　著作権法上、無断複写・複製は禁じられています。

Oliver Sacks' *Awakenings*		[B-813]
『レナードの朝』で学ぶ医療問題とクリティカル・シンキング			

1　刷	2016年 1 月 15 日
5　刷	2025年 3 月 21 日

原著者	Oliver Sacks　　オリバー・サックス
編著者	平井　清子　　Seiko Hirai

発行者	南雲　一範　Kazunori Nagumo
発行所	株式会社　南雲堂 〒 162-0801　東京都新宿区山吹町 361 NAN'UN-DO CO.,Ltd. 361 Yamabuki-cho, Shinjuku-ku, Tokyo 162-0801, Japan 振替口座：00160-0-46863 TEL：03-3268-2311 (代表)／FAX：03-3269-2486
印刷所	倉敷印刷（株）
検　印	省　略
コード	ISBN978-4-523-17813-2　　　　　　C0082

Printed in Japan

E-mail　　nanundo@post.email.ne.jp
URL　　　https://www.nanun-do.co.jp/

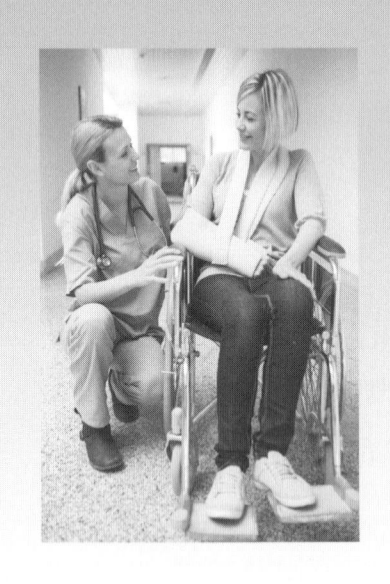

英和対訳

実践 看護の英会話

四六判 CD付 256ページ 定価（本体 1,900円＋税）

西村月満・平井清子・和治元義博 訳

世界最大規模の医学系出版社エルゼビア社の『Everyday English for International Nurses (Joy Parkinson/Chris Brooker)』の対訳本です。見開きで英文と日本文を掲載。現場で役立つ会話部分は添付のCDに完全収録（MP3）！ 教育現場で効果実践済みの語学書です。

南雲堂